DISEASES AND DISORDERS

SKIN CANCER

AMERICA'S MOST COMMON CANCER

By Peter Kogler

Portions of this book originally appeared in *Skin Cancer* by Bonnie Juettner.

LUCENT
PRESS

Published in 2019 by
Lucent Press, an Imprint of Greenhaven Publishing, LLC
353 3rd Avenue
Suite 255
New York, NY 10010

Designer: Andrea Davison-Bartolotta
Editor: Jennifer Lombardo

Library of Congress Cataloging-in-Publication Data

Names: Kogler, Peter, author.
Title: Skin cancer : America's most common cancer / Peter Kogler.
Description: New York : Lucent, 2019. | Series: Diseases and disorders | Includes bibliographical references and index.
Identifiers: LCCN 2018020768 (print) | LCCN 2018022428 (ebook) | ISBN 9781534564909 (eBook) | ISBN 9781534564893 (library bound book) | ISBN 9781534564886 (pbk. book)
Subjects: LCSH: Skin—Cancer—United States.
Classification: LCC RC280.S5 (ebook) | LCC RC280.S5 K64 2019 (print) | DDC 616.99/477—dc23
LC record available at https://lccn.loc.gov/2018020768

Printed in the United States of America

CPSIA compliance information: Batch #BW19KL: For further information contact Greenhaven Publishing LLC, New York, New York, at 1-844-317-7404.

Please visit our website, www.greenhavenpublishing.com. For a free color catalog of all our high-quality books, call toll free 1-844-317-7404 or fax 1-844-317-7405.

CONTENTS

FOREWORD

Illness is an unfortunate part of life, and it is one that is often misunderstood. Thanks to advances in science and technology, people have been aware for many years that diseases such as the flu, pneumonia, and chicken pox are caused by viruses and bacteria. These diseases all cause physical symptoms that people can see and understand, and many people have dealt with these diseases themselves. However, sometimes diseases that were previously unknown in most of the world turn into epidemics and spread across the globe. Without an awareness of the method by which these diseases are spread—through the air, through human waste or fluids, through sexual contact, or by some other method—people cannot take the proper precautions to prevent further contamination. Panic often accompanies epidemics as a result of this lack of knowledge.

Knowledge is power in the case of mental disorders, as well. Mental disorders are just as common as physical disorders, but due to a lack of awareness among the general public, they are often stigmatized. Scientists have studied them for years and have found that they are generally caused by hormonal imbalances in the brain, but they have not yet determined with certainty what causes those imbalances or how to fix them. Because even mild mental illness is stigmatized in Western society, many people prefer not to talk about it.

Chronic pain disorders are also not well understood—even by researchers—and do not yet have foolproof treatments. People who have a mental disorder or a disease or disorder that causes them to feel chronic pain can be the target of uninformed opinions. People who do not have these disorders sometimes struggle to understand how difficult it can be to deal with the symptoms. These disorders are often termed "invisible illnesses" because no one can see the symptoms; this leads many people to doubt that they exist or are serious problems. Additionally, people who have an undiagnosed disorder may understand that they are experiencing the world in a different way than their peers, but they have no one to turn to for answers.

Misinformation about all kinds of ailments is often spread through personal anecdotes, social media, and even news sources. This series aims to present accurate information about both physical and mental conditions so young adults will have a better understanding of them. Each volume discusses the symptoms of a particular disease or disorder, ways it is currently being treated, and the research that is being done to understand it further. Advice for people who may be suffering from the disorder is included, as well as information for their loved ones about how best to support them.

With fully cited quotes, a list of recommended books and websites for further research, and informational charts, this series provides young adults with a factual introduction to common illnesses. By learning more about these ailments, they will be better able to prevent the spread of contagious diseases, show compassion to people who are dealing with invisible illnesses, and take charge of their own health.

INTRODUCTION

THINKING TWICE ABOUT THE SUN

In the United States alone, more than 5 million people are treated for skin cancer each year, with an economic cost of more than $8 billion. Melanoma—now considered the most dangerous type of skin cancer—is currently one of the most common types of cancer among teenagers and young adults, but at one time, it was a rare disease. As skin cancer rates in general continue to rise, dermatologists have found this increase to be alarming.

According to the Skin Cancer Foundation, melanoma will kill about 9,320 Americans in 2018. Skin cancer rates are climbing steadily, which means health care costs are increasing as well. In the words of Dr. Joseph Sobanko, "If you add up all of the non-melanoma skin cancers each year, that number is greater than all of the new cases of breast, prostate, colon, lung, and melanoma skin cancers combined."[1]

There is an overwhelmingly strong correlation between skin cancer and the ultraviolet (UV) rays that people are exposed to daily from the sun. Prevention education has been found to be successful in reducing skin cancer cases, but there is still a long way to go.

Resisting That Tan

Dermatologists believe the increase in melanomas is partly the result of changing social attitudes. Pale skin used to be fashionable; it was a way of proving that

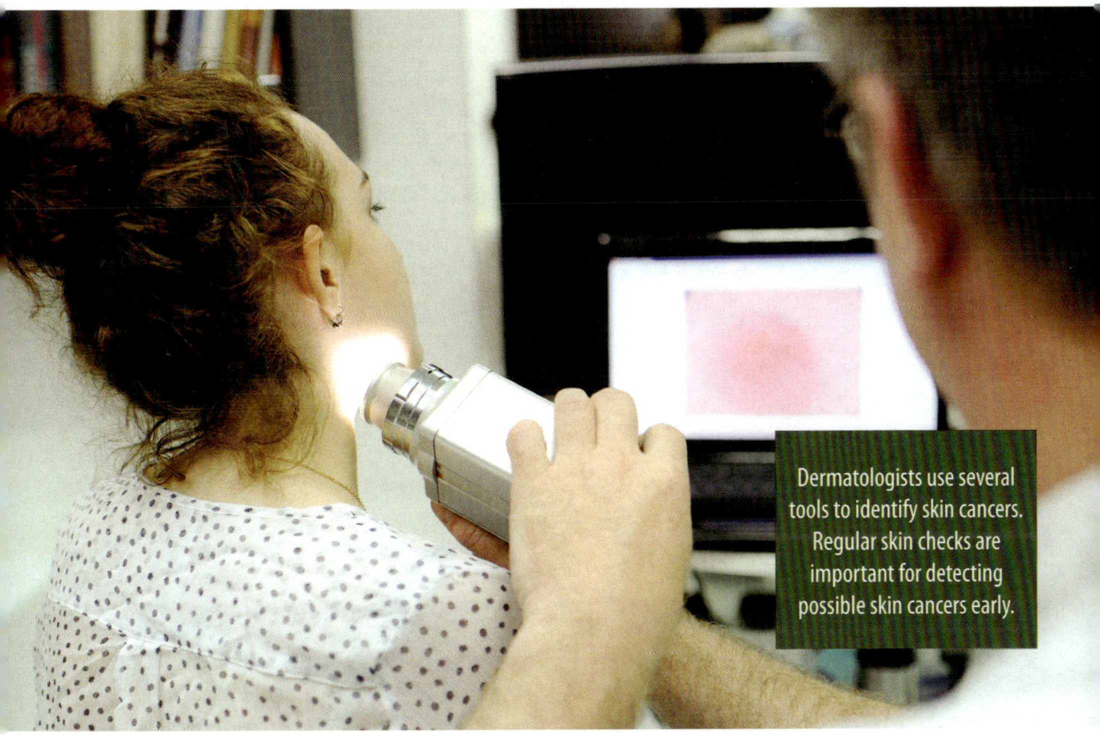

Dermatologists use several tools to identify skin cancers. Regular skin checks are important for detecting possible skin cancers early.

one was a member of the upper class. Those who did have tans were lower-class people who worked outside, such as farmers, construction workers, and shipyard workers. In 2009, a group of researchers examined early 20th-century magazines and discovered that tanning became fashionable somewhere between the 1920s and 1930s. During this time, people began to view a tan as a sign of good health.

Many myths persist about the relationship between sun and skin. For instance, although most people know that sunburn increases the risk of developing skin cancer, some believe that getting a tan will prevent the skin from burning later. However, in June 2017, the Mayo Clinic debunked this myth, saying, "There's little evidence to support the idea that a base tan protects you against sunburn."[2] According to the American Cancer Society, "Whether tanning or burning, you are exposing yourself to harmful UV rays that damage your skin. In fact, every time you tan, you increase your risk of melanoma."[3] Indoor tanning is considered so bad for a person's health that federal, state, and local governments are pushing for laws protecting people under 18 years old by banning them from using tanning beds. In 2017, the American Academy of Pediatrics reported that 17 states and Washington, D.C., had these laws. If a person does decide to get a tan, they should take the advice of the American Academy of Dermatology, which says, "If you want to look tan, use a self-tanning product, but continue using sunscreen with it."[4] Self-tanning products are creams and lotions that make the skin look tan without exposing someone to UV rays.

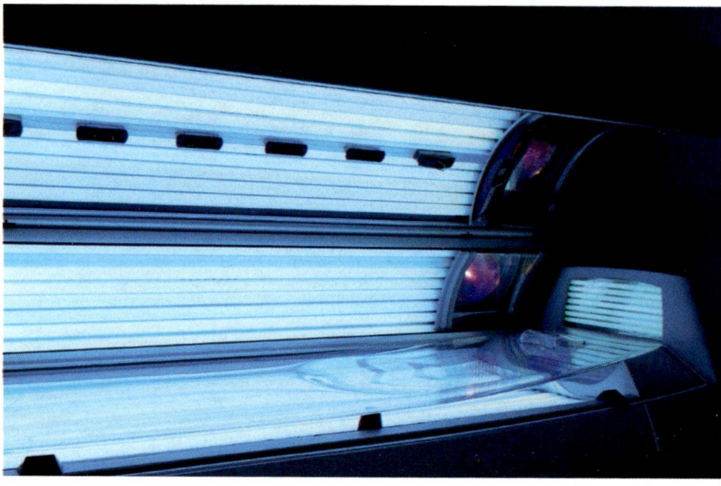

Recent laws have made it more difficult for young teens to use tanning beds similar to this one. The UV rays from tanning beds are just as dangerous as UV rays from the sun.

Sunburn and Melanoma

Tanning and sunburns are even more dangerous for children and teenagers than for adults. Dermatologists believe most skin cancers begin in childhood. Part of the problem is that children and teens spend much more time in the sun than adults do. In fact, the World Health Organization (WHO) estimates that "up to 80 percent of a person's lifetime exposure to UV is received before the age of 18."[5] In January 2018, the Skin Cancer Foundation reported, "On average, a person's risk for melanoma doubles if he or she has had more than five sunburns."[6] Fortunately, sunburn is easily preventable with a few precautions.

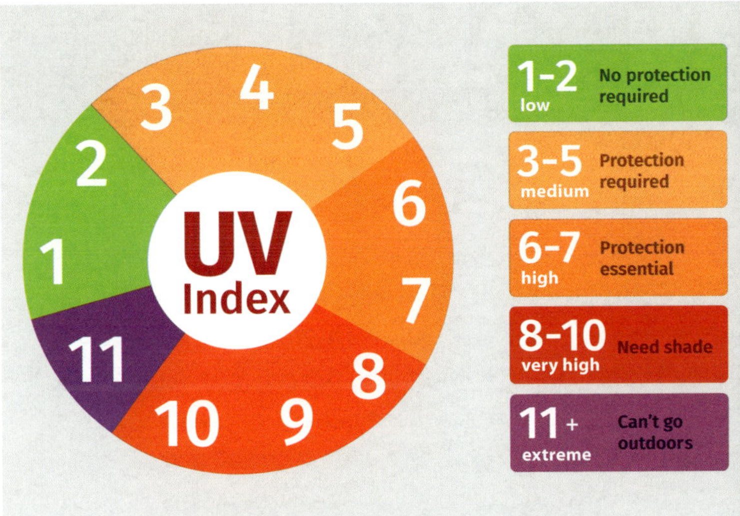

The UV index scale is designed to give the public an idea of how strong UV rays will be on a given day. The Environmental Protection Agency (EPA) recommends the use of sunscreen and sunglasses even at the lowest UV index levels.

Detecting Skin Cancer Early

Skin cancer of all types can be deadly, and melanoma is one of the deadliest. The Skin Cancer Foundation reported in 2018 that melanoma kills one person every hour and estimated that 5,990 men and 3,330 women would die from melanoma that year. There is good news, however. Self-exams and doctor's visits can lead to what is called "early detection." Both non-melanoma and melanoma skin cancer can be successfully treated if they are detected early enough.

As Doctor H. William Higgins explained, "The earliest form of melanoma (considered stage 0) … is the easiest to treat and almost always curable."[7] When skin cancer is detected and treated early, a person has a 99 percent survival rate. The longer it goes undetected and treated, the lower that survival rate becomes. This makes recognizing skin cancer and getting regular checkups extremely important.

CHAPTER ONE

DEFINING SKIN CANCER

There are multiple types of skin cancer, and many people are not familiar with all of them. This can make identifying cancer tricky. It is important to know the warning signs of any skin cancer because, like other cancers, skin cancer is easier to treat if it is detected early. The survival rate for skin cancer is actually higher than that for other cancers, such as lung cancer or breast cancer. Also, because skin cancer develops visibly on the skin, a person has a better chance of finding it early.

How Sunlight Changes DNA

Skin cancer, like other kinds of cancer, is caused by mutations in a cell's deoxyribonucleic acid (DNA). A cell's DNA is like a blueprint that tells it how to reproduce itself exactly. When the DNA is damaged, cells can mutate. A small percentage of mutations occur randomly and have no particular cause. More commonly, however, mutations are caused by mutagens, which are physical or chemical agents that can damage DNA. The UV radiation in sunlight is a mutagen that can cause healthy skin cells to produce mutant skin cells.

When skin cells are damaged, they do not know how to work properly. They begin to multiply at an

The Skin's Many Functions

The skin covers the entire body, making up about one-seventh of a person's body weight. The skin helps protect the body from invasion by viruses or bacteria. It controls the amount of heat the body gives off, helping to keep the body from getting too hot or cold by regulating temperature. It also contains nerve endings that send the brain important information about the body's environment and gives someone their sense of touch.

The skin also:

- protects the inner organs
- blocks UV radiation
- kills bacteria
- holds in moisture
- repairs small cuts and burns

Because the skin has so many important functions, it is important that a person takes steps to protect it on a daily basis. Damaged skin cannot do its many jobs effectively.

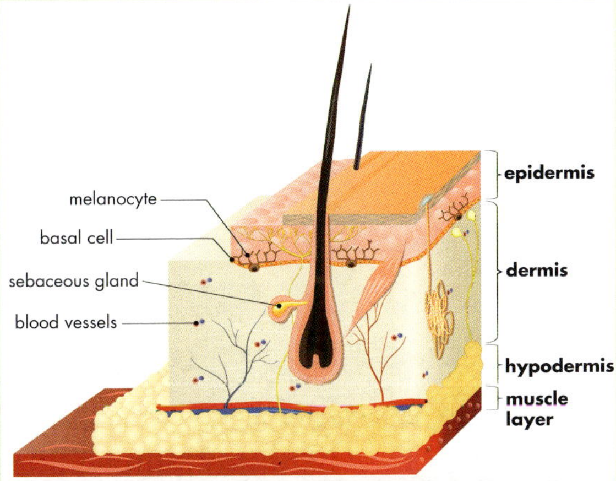

The skin has multiple layers, each of which serve an important function.

accelerated rate, forming tumors, which are groups of mutated cells. Some tumors are not dangerous; these are called benign tumors. When they are life-threatening, they are known as malignant tumors. Cancer that stays on the surface of the skin—the layer called the epidermis—is generally not fatal because it can easily be removed. However, skin cancer, even in the early stages, is serious because it can spread. If it invades a lymph node, it can travel through the lymphatic system, which carries fluid throughout the body. This, unfortunately, allows cancer cells to travel to organs of the body that might be far away from the original cancer site.

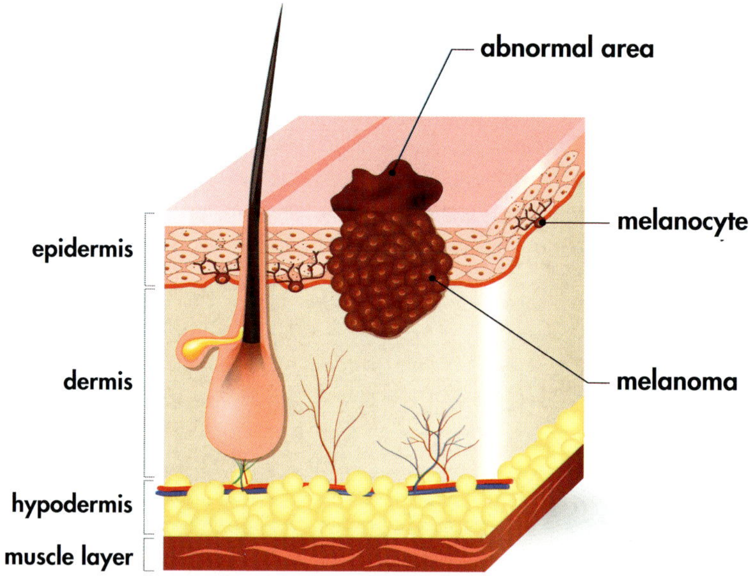

The longer skin cancer goes untreated, the more difficult it is to remove. Once cancer spreads deeper into the layers of the skin, as shown here, it can be much more difficult to treat.

Three Cells, Three Cancers

There are three types of skin cancer. Just as cancers are named according to the organ on which they first develop, types of skin cancer are named after the type of skin cell they mutate from. The outer layer of the skin is called the epidermis. It contains three kinds of cells. The top layer of the epidermis is made up of flat, scaly cells, called squamous cells. The epidermis also contains melanocytes, which are cells that give a person their skin color. Underneath these lie the third type of cells, known as basal cells.

Cancer that develops from the skin's basal cells is not only the most common type of skin cancer but also the most common of any cancer. The medical term for skin cancer is "carcinoma." The Skin Cancer Foundation reported in 2018 that in the United States, more than 4 million cases of basal cell carcinoma are diagnosed each year. Generally, these cancers appear on the face, neck, or hands. Fortunately, most basal cell carcinomas are not fatal and are very often easy to treat. According to dermatologist Gregory L. Wells,

> *Basal cell carcinomas rarely spread (metastasize) to other parts of the body. Instead, they invade and slowly destroy surrounding tissues. When basal cell carcinomas grow near the eyes, ears, mouth, bone, or brain, the consequences of spread can be serious and can lead to death. Yet, for most people, the tumors simply grow slowly into the skin.*[8]

Cancer that develops from the skin's squamous cells is called squamous cell carcinoma. Squamous cell cancers are the second most common form of skin cancer. When they are detected early, they are also easy to cure. However, if left untreated, they tend to spread to nearby lymph nodes, where they can be deadly.

Malignant melanoma is a cancer that develops out of a melanocyte. It is the least common but most life-threatening form of skin cancer. Melanomas can quickly spread to other parts of the body, where they can invade other organs, such as the brain, liver, or stomach. When cancer spreads this way, it is called metastatic. Fortunately, it is not difficult to detect melanomas, and it is easy to reduce the risk that they will develop in the first place.

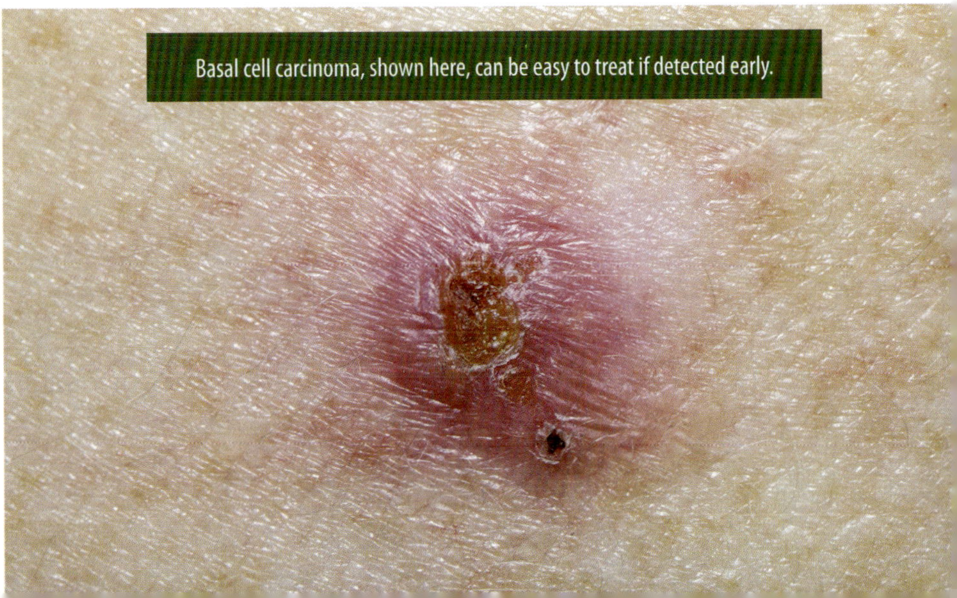

Basal cell carcinoma, shown here, can be easy to treat if detected early.

The Shadow Rule

Some people may think of sunscreen as the only line of defense against sunburn. However, there are other precautions that people can take. Dawn Holman, a behavioral scientist for the Centers for Disease Control and Prevention (CDC), explained,

> *Using sunscreen can reduce your risk of skin cancer and early skin aging, but it shouldn't be your only line of defense against the sun ... It's best to combine sunscreen with other forms of sun protection. Communities can help with strategies like providing shade in outdoor areas, which can make it easier for individuals to stay sun-safe while enjoying the outdoors.*[9]

UV ray intensity is directly affected by the angle of the sun and the sun's altitude, or height, in the sky. The American Skin Association recommends following something called the "shadow rule": When a person's shadow is shorter than the person is, it means the sun's UV rays are at their most intense—and most damaging. When this happens, a person should find some shade or get indoors in order to avoid the most serious UV damage.

More Than Fashion

Damage from sunlight can occur in less than 15 minutes. Therefore, many dermatologists recommend dressing appropriately for the sun, which includes wearing a hat. According to the CDC,

> *For the most protection, wear a hat with a brim all the way around that shades your face, ears, and the back of your neck ... Avoid straw hats with holes that let sunlight through. A darker hat may offer more UV protection. If you wear a baseball cap, you should also protect your ears and the back of your neck by wearing clothing that covers those*

areas, using a broad spectrum sunscreen with at least SPF 15, or by staying in the shade.[10]

The clothes that people wear are important, too. While long-sleeve shirts and pants are the best protection, this is not always practical or comfortable on a hot day. A simple T-shirt is better than nothing, but it is still important to use sunscreen. Eyes also need to be protected, as UV rays can damage the lens and cornea, leading to cataracts—clouding of the lens, which interferes with vision—in the future. Sunglasses with UV protective lenses will block anywhere from 99 to 100 percent of dangerous rays.

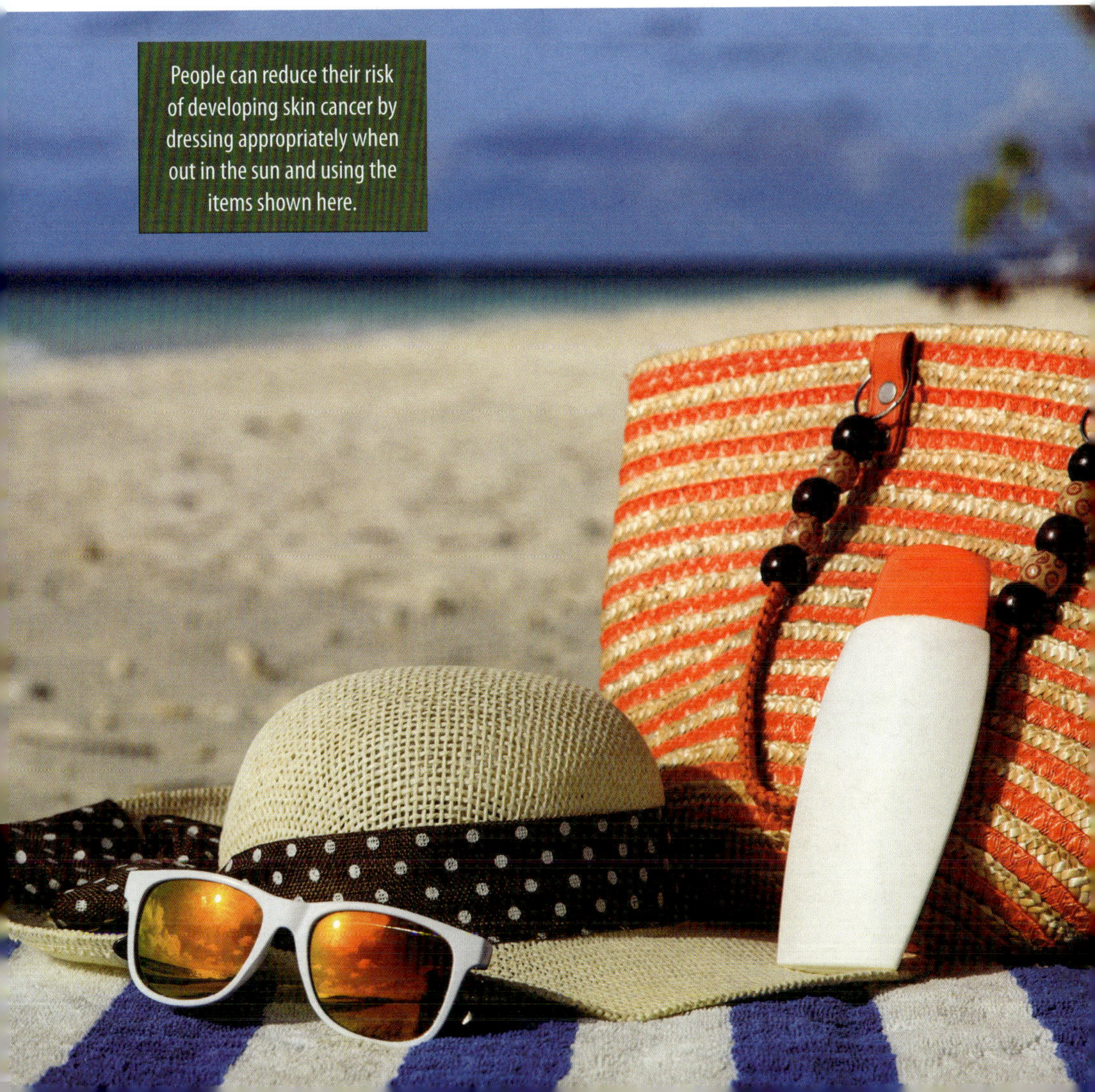

People can reduce their risk of developing skin cancer by dressing appropriately when out in the sun and using the items shown here.

Getting the Most Out of Sunscreen

In a 2013 survey, the CDC discovered that sunscreen is used less by lower-income families and non-Hispanic black people who have skin that is less sensitive to UV rays. In fact, that survey showed just how many people in general fall short when it comes to using sunscreen. The CDC reported, "Only 14.3 percent of men and 29.9 percent of women reported that they regularly use sunscreen on both their face and other exposed skin."[11]

The Skin Cancer Foundation recommends that people use an ounce of sunscreen—which amounts to about two tablespoons—to cover their bodies. It is not a good idea to apply the first coat of sunscreen outside. Instead, it should be applied at least 30 minutes before sun exposure and then reapplied every 2 hours outdoors. Pre-applying sunscreen allows the skin to absorb it properly. If a person is swimming or sweating, sunscreen should be reapplied immediately, as it washes away.

People Still Need Some Sun

While prolonged sun exposure is dangerous, the sun is actually essential for people. It is healthy to spend some time in the sun every day. Sunlight stimulates the body to produce vitamin D, which has many important functions, such as bone growth in people of all ages. Too little vitamin D "has now been linked to breast cancer, colon cancer, prostate cancer, heart disease, depression, weight gain, and other maladies."[12] The key here is that a person does not need much sun exposure to produce vitamin D. As reported by the Skin Cancer Foundation in 2016, "no more than 10 to 15 minutes of exposure to arms, legs, abdomen and back, two to three times a week, followed by good sun protection"[13] will do the trick.

Since absorbing UV rays is essential to vitamin D creation and sunscreen blocks those rays, theoretically, using sunscreen should interfere with the body's production of the vitamin. Experts are divided on this matter. One Australian study compared the vitamin D levels between groups using sunscreen and a placebo, or fake, sunscreen. The study found that there was no difference in vitamin D levels between the two groups at the end of the study. However, some say this may be because the sunscreen was applied improperly or not frequently enough. Another study found that when a sunscreen with an SPF of 15 or more is properly applied, it can reduce the production of vitamin D by up to 99 percent. However, the 10 to 15 minutes of sun exposure needed to get enough vitamin D is not enough time for UV rays to damage the skin, so there is little to no danger from being outside for a few minutes without sunscreen. It should always be used if someone is planning to be outside for a longer period of time.

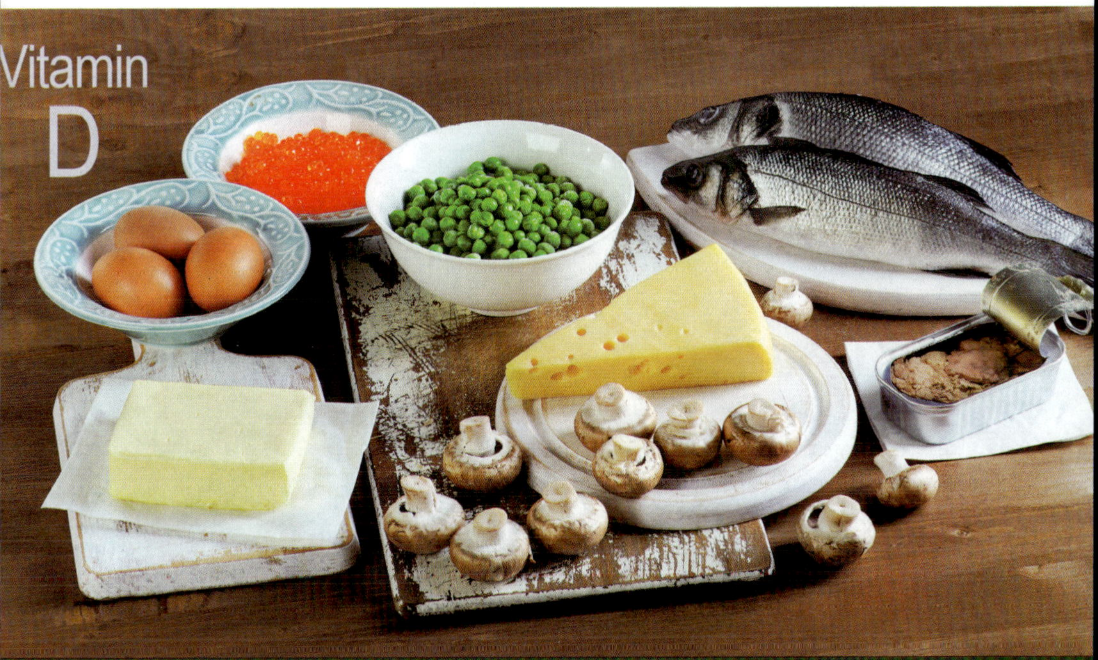

People do not get all of their vitamin D from the sun. In fact, they can get it through eating vitamin D–rich foods, such as tuna, salmon, egg yolks, cheese, and certain vegetables.

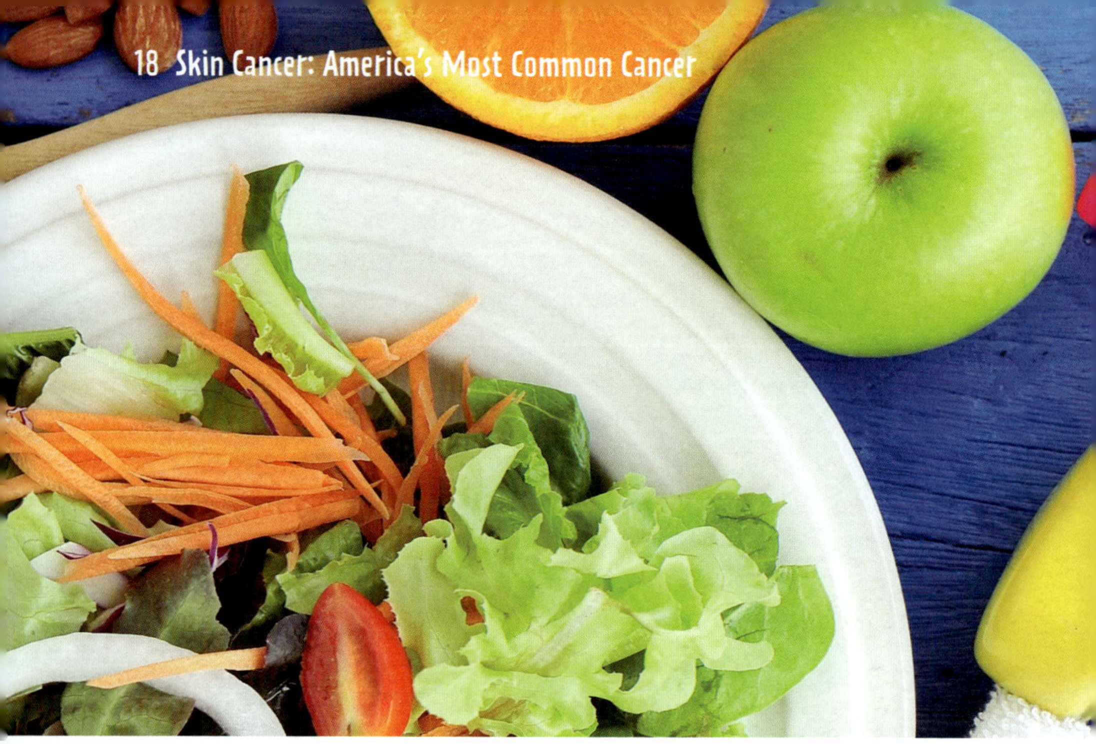

A Delicious Finding

The best ways to prevent skin cancer are to avoid being out in the sun, covering the skin, and wearing good sunscreen. However, some researchers have discovered that cocoa beans—a key ingredient in chocolate—have some interesting UV-blocking properties. In 2009, researchers did a study in which they had 30 participants eat a small piece of chocolate for 12 weeks as a mid-morning snack. One group ate chocolate that was rich with flavonols, while the other group did not.

Flavonols are a class of flavonoids. Flavonoids, which are chemicals found in most vegetables and fruits, are believed to have beneficial health effects. They also help give fruits and vegetables their bright colors. Conventional chocolate making uses high heat that destroys flavonol, so for this study, specially prepared chocolate was created for the group that needed to consume the flavonols. The researchers then used a special UV light on the participants' forearms to determine which dose of UV rays would create sunburn.

At the end of the 12 weeks, those who consumed the flavonol-rich chocolate could withstand double the amount of UV rays without getting sunburned. Apples, green tea, citrus fruits, berries, and many other foods are also rich in flavonoids, and ongoing studies will continue to research these UV-protecting effects. However, it is important to note that eating chocolate or any other flavonol-rich food is not a substitute for using sunscreen, especially if someone is outside in strong sunlight for several hours.

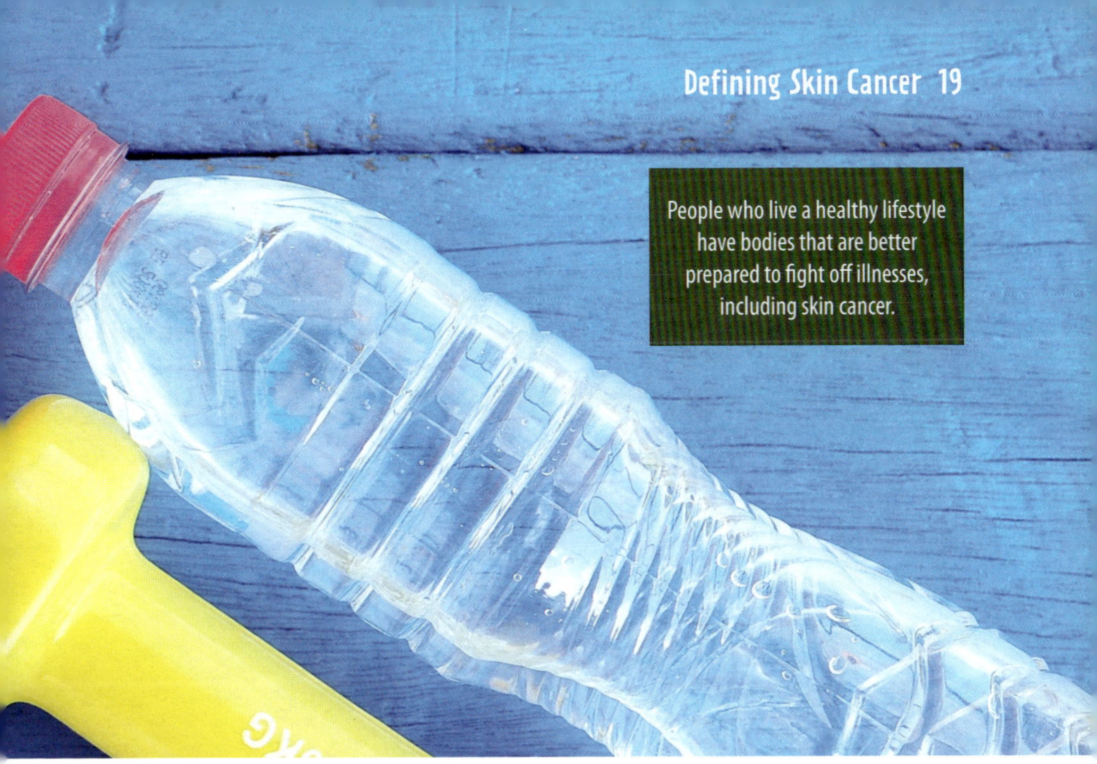

People who live a healthy lifestyle have bodies that are better prepared to fight off illnesses, including skin cancer.

Healthy Body, Healthy Life

According to the American Cancer Society, "Research has shown that poor diet and not being active are two key factors that can increase a person's cancer risk."[14] To reduce their risk of skin cancer, people should be eating plenty of fresh fruits and vegetables, exercising, getting plenty of rest, and most of all, covering up skin that is exposed to the sun. A healthy lifestyle cannot guarantee that a person will never develop skin cancer, but a healthy body can more easily recover from an unexpected shock—even if that shock happens to be skin cancer.

CHAPTER TWO

A GROWING CAUSE FOR CONCERN

The American Academy of Dermatology estimates that 9,500 Americans are diagnosed with skin cancer every day, with approximately 178,560 new melanoma cases expected in 2018 alone. The WHO estimates that there are 65,000 melanoma-related deaths worldwide every year. However, doctors say that all melanoma deaths are preventable. Like other cancers, if skin cancer is detected early enough, removal and treatment can occur. The longer it is left untreated, the less likely it is to be cured.

The Role of Genetics

Skin cancer does not strike people randomly. In fact, some people are more at risk than others. The biggest risk factor is spending a lot of time in the sun without taking proper precautions. Sunlight does not affect everyone in exactly the same way, as there are many differing factors. For instance, race plays a role because of the difference in skin color, which is related to the amount of melanocytes a person has in their skin. According to the American Cancer Society (ACS), "the lifetime risk of getting melanoma is about 2.6% (1 in 38) for whites, 0.1% (1 in 1,000) for blacks, and 0.58% (1 in 172) for Hispanics."[15]

Those with fair skin tend to get sunburned more easily, and people with blonde or red hair, green or blue eyes, and freckles have a higher risk of developing skin cancer. This is because of the genes that are tied to those traits. Genes contain the information that determines things such as a person's eye color and risk of certain diseases. Multiple genes are involved in most traits, and sometimes they are linked in ways that are not immediately obvious. For unknown reasons, the genes that determine blue eyes and red hair and the genes that determine how likely a person's skin is to be damaged by the sun are connected. Family history, such as a parent or grandparent who had skin cancer, can also increase a person's risk. Personal history, such as previous sunburns, tanning bed usage, and even the presence of many large moles (which are groups of melanocytes that create a dark spot on the skin) can also greatly increase the chances of skin cancer.

Dark-skinned people have more melanin—the chemical produced by melanocytes—in their skin, which reduces their risk of skin cancer. This is because melanin acts as a sort of natural sunscreen. Dark skin is a trait that developed thousands of years ago in people who lived in very sunny climates, such as Africa, India, and South America. Before the invention of sunscreen, people who lived in these places needed a natural way for their bodies to protect them from the sun's UV rays. However, melanin protects skin only up to a certain point, so people with dark skin are not immune to skin cancer. Dr. Maritza Perez pointed out that "many people of color are less susceptible to UV damage thanks to the greater amounts of melanin (the protective pigment that gives skin and eyes their color) darker skin produces. But people of color can still develop skin cancer from UV damage."[16] Other studies have found similar results. Additionally, a 2016 study found that although patients of color were less likely to develop melanoma compared to Caucasian patients, they were also less likely to survive it after they developed it.

The Role of Personal and Family History

Dermatologists generally begin a skin cancer screening by learning about a person's medical history, which can reveal if a person is at greater risk for cancer. This history will look at previous sun and tanning bed exposure as well as a background of the patient's family members. People who have family members with skin cancer are more likely to develop it themselves. According to the National Cancer Institute, "About 10 percent of all patients with melanoma have another family member with this disease; only about 1% of individuals with melanoma have more than one family member with melanoma."[17]

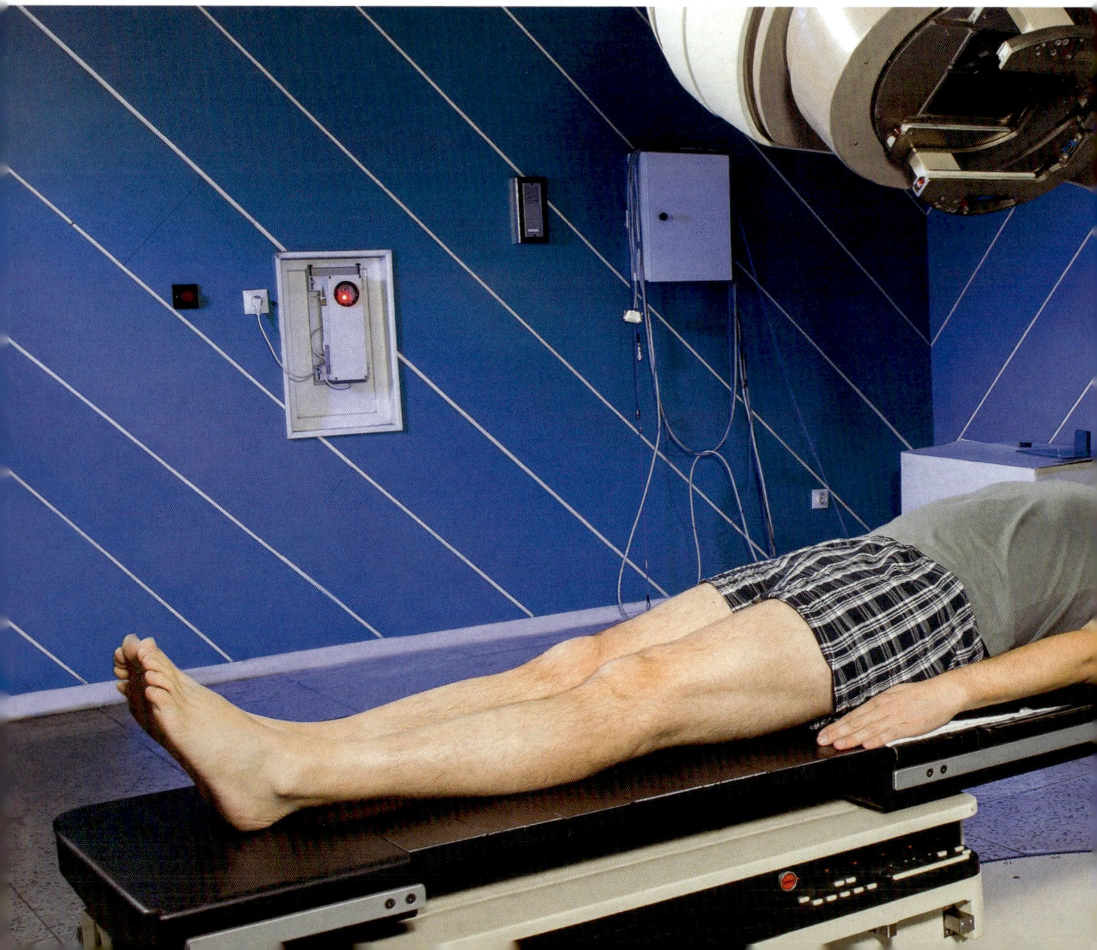

Individuals who have had skin cancer before are also more at risk to develop it again, although they may not necessarily develop the same exact kind. For example, a survivor of basal cell carcinoma is at greater than average risk for developing squamous cell carcinoma or melanoma, not just other basal cell cancers. Other aspects of their medical history can also increase a person's risk for skin cancer. In the 1930s, dermatologists treated acne with radiation. People who had radiation treatment for acne when they were teenagers often developed skin cancer as adults. The ACS says, "People who have had radiation treatment have a higher risk of developing skin cancer in the area that received the treatment. This is particularly a concern in children who have had radiation treatment for cancer."[18]

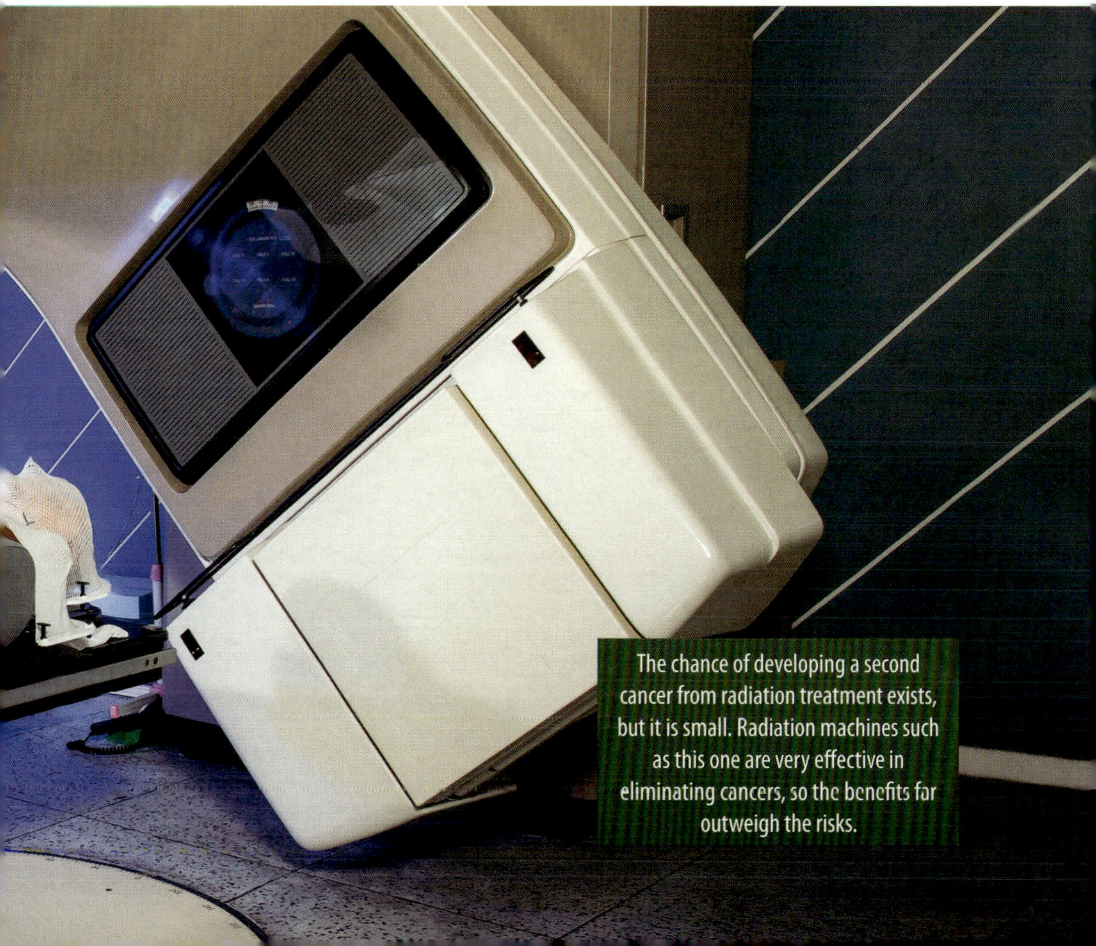

The chance of developing a second cancer from radiation treatment exists, but it is small. Radiation machines such as this one are very effective in eliminating cancers, so the benefits far outweigh the risks.

The Role of Location and Other Factors

Living in a part of the world that is close to the equator, where the sun is more intense, also increases risk, even for people who do not like to go tanning. In March 2016, researchers from the QIMR Berghofer Medical Research Institute found that New Zealand had the highest melanoma rates in the world, surpassing Australia for the first time. The Cancer Center of Australia reported, "Approximately, two in three Australians will be diagnosed with skin cancer by the time they are 70, with more than 750,000 people treated for one or more non-melanoma skin cancers in Australia each year."[19]

The reason New Zealand and Australia have the highest melanoma rates in the world may largely have to do with the fact that they are located close to the equator. Furthermore, the ancestors of many people who currently live in New Zealand and Australia largely came from the British Isles and had fair skin that was more susceptible to damaging UV rays. The people who had lived in New Zealand and Australia for years before the British arrived and took over—much the same way they did in what is now the United States—have more melanin in their skin because their bodies evolved to protect them from the sun. They have a lower rate of skin cancer than light-skinned Australians and New Zealanders, whose ancestors' skin evolved to maximize the amount of vitamin D it could absorb in places where the sun is less intense, such as England.

Some risk factors for skin cancer may be surprising because they do not seem to be related to the skin. People who have had organ transplants have a greater risk because they take immune system–suppressing drugs to ensure that their body does not attack the new organ. However, this means that their bodies are weaker and less able to effectively fight skin cancer. The same can be said of those suffering from HIV and AIDS because they also have weakened immune systems. The ACS reported, "Workers exposed to coal tar, paraffin, and certain types of oil may also have an increased risk of skin cancer."[20]

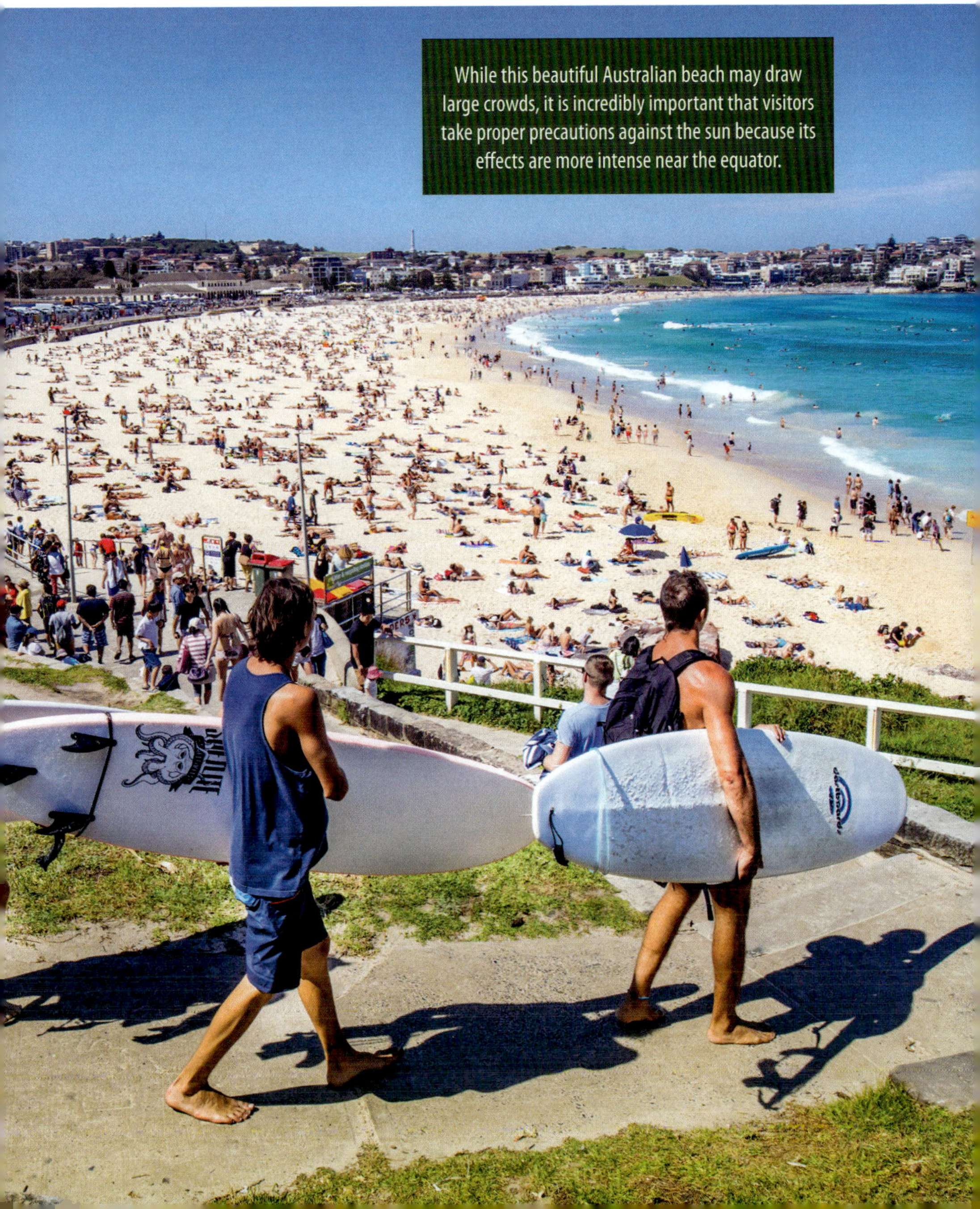

While this beautiful Australian beach may draw large crowds, it is incredibly important that visitors take proper precautions against the sun because its effects are more intense near the equator.

An Unequal Focus

According to studies, women are more likely to get skin cancer, but men are more likely to die from it. In 2012, the Skin Cancer Foundation created a survey to judge men's use of sunblock and skin cancer awareness. The survey results revealed "that nearly half (49%) of men in the US [admitted] to not using sunscreen in the past 12 months and an alarming 70 percent of men [did not] even know what skin cancer warning signs to look for."[1] In 2013, the organization also estimated that of the 9,480 people who died from melanoma that year in the United States, nearly two-thirds were men.

The Skin Cancer Foundation's research did not end there. In 2014, it reported why men are less likely to detect skin cancer early. The researchers looked at biological factors, behavioral factors, and even the socio-economic status of the study group. They found that "most of the recent public health messages regarding tanning bed and suntan avoidance have focused on women."[2] Men, therefore, were not being properly educated on sun precautions and early screening techniques. The researchers advised, "Men of all ages should seek prompt [quick] medical attention for any changing moles or skin lesions that look different from the rest."[3] This early detection can save lives.

1. "New Survey Reveals Gender Divide Surrounding Skin Cancer Awareness and Prevention," Skin Cancer Foundation, June 20, 2012. www.skincancer.org/media-and-press/press-release-2012/survey.

2. Susan M. Swetter, Christina A. Clarke, and Theresa H. M. Keegan, "Why Do Men Have Worse Melanoma Survival than Women? Is It Behavior, Biology, or Both?," Skin Cancer Foundation, *The Melanoma Letter*, vol. 32, no. 2, Summer 2014. www.skincancer.org/publications/the-melanoma-letter/summer-2014-vol-32-no-2/men.

3. Swetter, Clarke, and Keegan, "Why Do Men Have Worse Melanoma Survival than Women?"

ABCDE and the Five Signs

Detecting skin cancer early means a higher chance of survival. Because skin lies on the surface of the body, it is relatively easy to detect skin cancer, even at home. Dermatologists recommend that people check their skin regularly by using a full-length mirror and a flashlight. It is important to check the back and the backs of the legs, even though it can be difficult to see them. To help people recognize the signs of early melanoma, dermatologists came up with the ABCDE test.

ABCDE stands for the five signs that a mole may be a melanoma. This acronym was created in 1985, although the letter E was not added until 2004. The letters represent the following:

- A stands for "asymmetry." Melanomas have irregular shapes and are not perfect circles.
- B stands for "border irregularity." Melanoma borders tend to look rough and broken.
- C stands for "color variation." Melanomas tend to be two or more shades, not one uniform color.
- D stands for "diameter." Melanomas do not look like tiny freckles. Instead, they tend to grow and reach diameters larger than five or six millimeters (a little less than a quarter of an inch).
- E stands for "evolving." Melanomas tend to change over time. For example, a mole may become darker in one area or expand to take up a larger area. Some moles grow and change their elevation. Moles that evolve should immediately be brought to the attention of a medical health professional.

Fortunately, most moles will pass the ABCDE test. Not all moles are melanomas, despite most moles being formed in response to the sun's UV radiation. Some people are even born with moles or have moles develop in places not exposed to the sun. All moles, however, have a risk of changing, and self-checks should be done once a month.

In 1998, French researchers introduced what is called the "ugly duckling test" to improve the ABCDE system for people who have multiple moles. If a patient has a group of moles that mostly pass the ABCDE test, then any abnormal "ugly duckling" ones will be easy to spot, since most benign moles in a cluster look similar to each other. In 2015, another group of French researchers put the ugly duckling method to the test. They were able to quickly and accurately find cancerous moles in both trials.

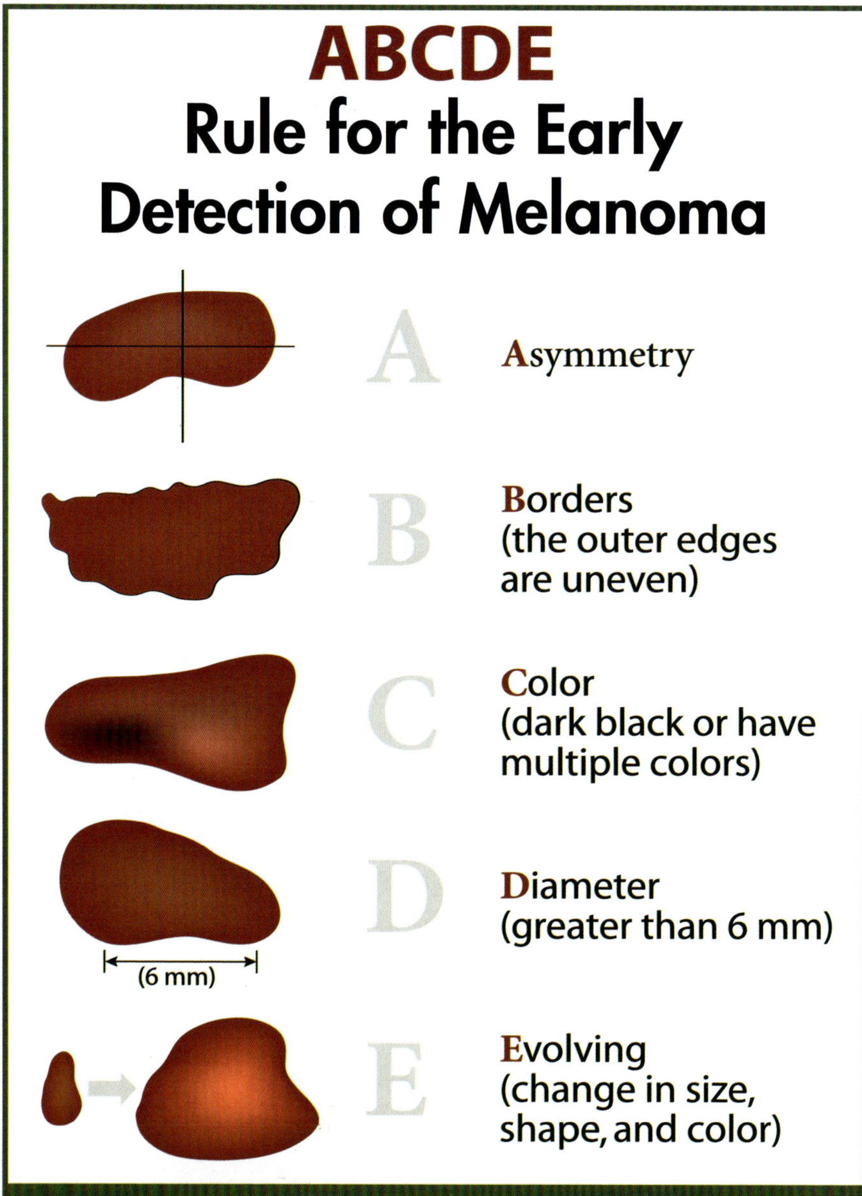

Charts such as this one might be posted in doctors' offices and hospitals. By learning the simple ABCDE system, people may be able to detect cancerous moles early—saving their lives in the process.

Skin Cancer–Detecting Apps?

In January 2017, Sebastian Thrun from the Stanford Artificial Intelligence Laboratory created a skin cancer–detecting program that may eventually become a skin cancer–detecting smartphone app. Using thousands of high-quality skin cancer images supplied by the University of Edinburgh and the International Skin Imaging Collaboration Project, Thrun and his team successfully created a computer algorithm that could correctly identify melanomas and carcinomas. In fact, the computer program's performance matched answers from a panel of 21 certified dermatologists.

Because smartphones are so widely used around the world, Thrun hopes this app will help many people in the future. Some similar apps, however, have been around for years. It is important to note that this technology can be inaccurate, as a 2012 study found. In 2013, the researchers of that study reported in *JAMA Dermatology* (a medical journal published by the American Medical Association) that "3 of 4 smartphone applications incorrectly classified 30% or more of melanomas as unconcerning."[1] As of 2018, nothing compares to a face-to-face exam with a real dermatologist. Someday, however, apps like these may become very important tools.

1. Joel A. Wolfe, "Diagnostic Inaccuracy of Smartphone Applications for Melanoma Detection," *JAMA Dermatology*, April 2013. jamanetwork.com/journals/jamadermatology/fullarticle/1557488?resultClick=3

A Dermatologist's Process

Skin that fails the ABCDE test needs to be checked by a dermatologist. A sore that does not heal can be a sign of cancer. An area of skin that is small, raised, smooth, shiny, and waxy can also be a sign. The opposite can apply, too, if a person has an area of skin that is flat, rough, and scaly. The growth on the skin might be red or reddish-brown, while some growths may bleed or become crusty. Other times, a growth can feel similar to a scar.

A dermatologist will ask about the area of skin itself. It is helpful to know when the mark first appeared and whether it has changed. Has it gotten bigger? Does it look different than it used to? Then, they use a special light and magnifying tool called a dermatoscope to examine the skin. Sometimes, dermatologists also check other areas of the skin to see if there are other marks similar to the one the person is concerned about and take pictures as needed. They may also check nearby lymph nodes to find out if they are swelling. If cancer has spread to the lymph nodes, they may be larger or firmer than usual. If the dermatologist suspects cancer, a biopsy from the affected area will be taken.

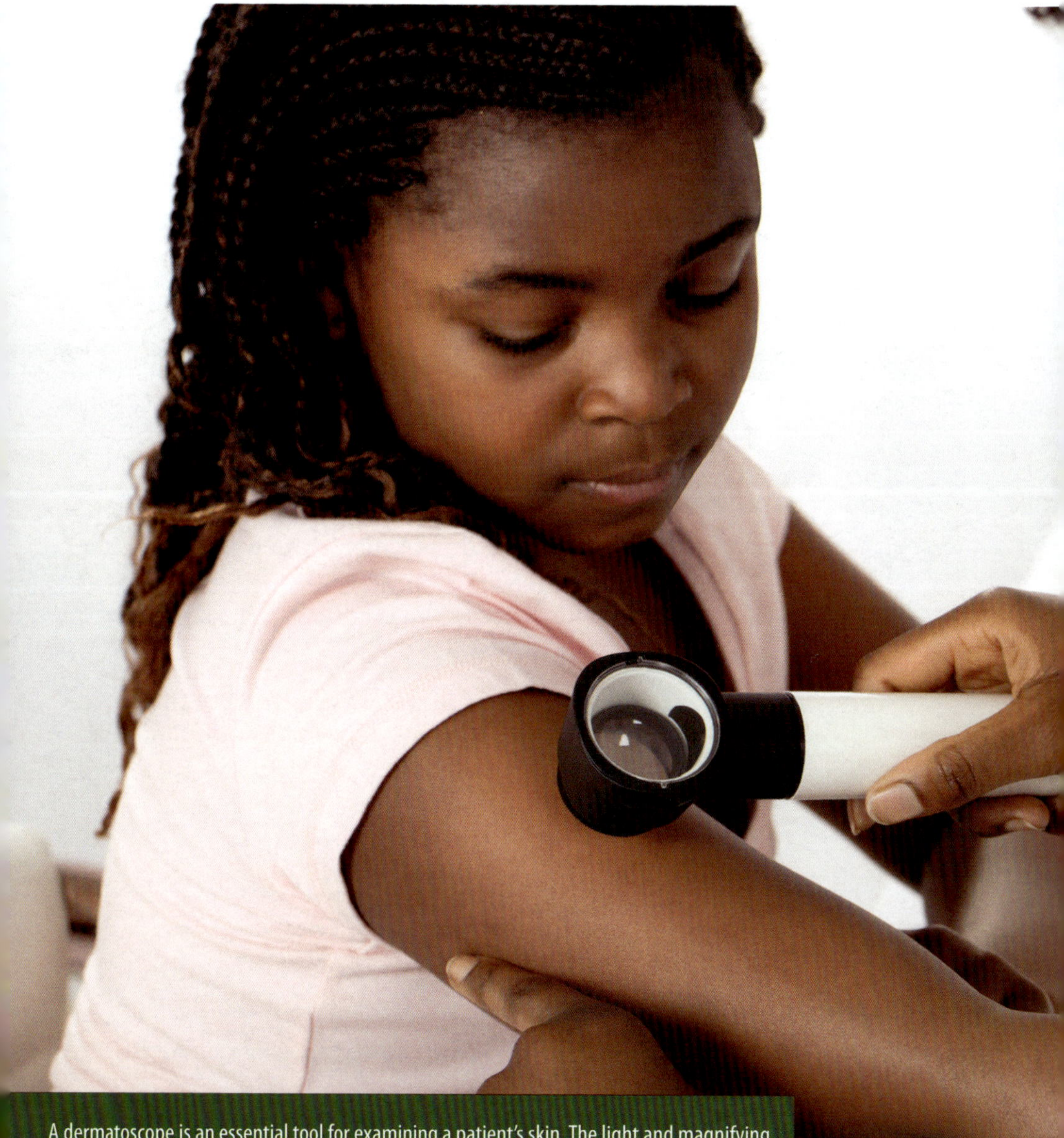

A dermatoscope is an essential tool for examining a patient's skin. The light and magnifying glass allow a doctor to see any troublesome spots up close and in great detail.

Biopsies of All Kinds

A biopsy is a kind of surgery in which the doctor cuts away a small sample of the skin. A pathologist will then examine the skin sample to determine whether or not any cancer cells are present. Pathologists are doctors who are trained to examine such tissue samples under a microscope. Sometimes, skin samples are sent to a dermatopathologist—a doctor who specializes in skin samples. There are many different types of biopsies, so doctors will choose the one that is best for the situation.

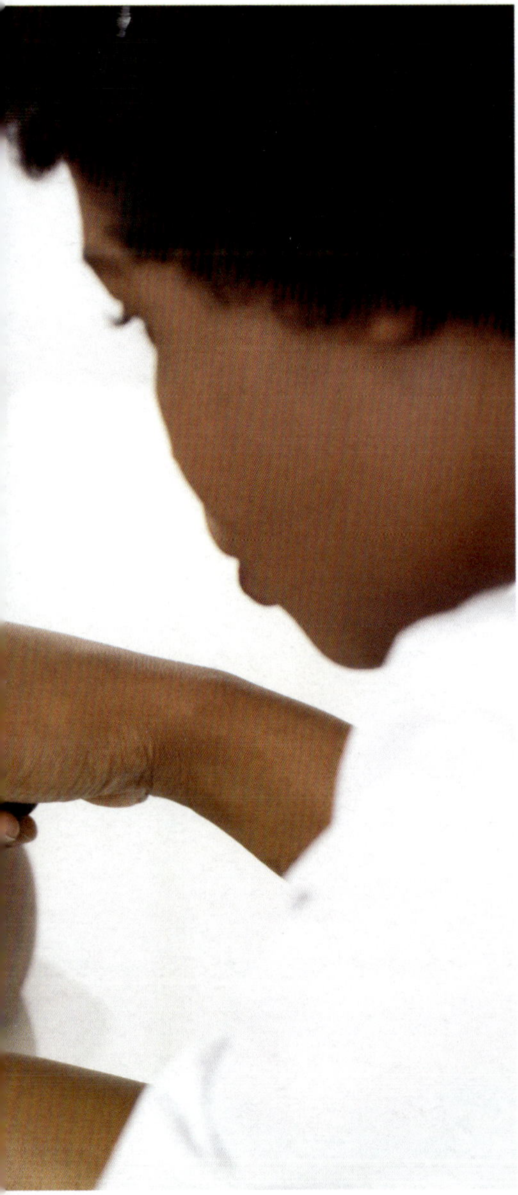

Former Olympic swimmer Summer Sanders explained how one biopsy led to others—which may have saved her life. "Right after my surgery [for one melanoma], I pointed out a faint spot on my other calf that was also fairly new," she said. "The doctor said he normally would not remove a spot like that, but since I said it started like the other one, he would take it off. Good thing we did, as the biopsy showed it was another melanoma, and caught early."[21] Another biopsy Sanders had in 2015 led to another diagnosis and removal.

Although a biopsy is a kind of surgery, it is relatively simple, and it can be done right in the dermatologist's office. Patients are given a local anesthetic, which numbs the skin where the biopsy will take place (as opposed to a general anesthetic, which puts them to sleep). Dermatologists can choose from several different types of biopsies, depending on how deeply they think a cancer may have penetrated the skin.

A shave biopsy takes layers of skin from the top, a punch biopsy uses a round cookie-cutter-like tool to remove the top layer of skin along with some deeper layers, and an incisional biopsy uses a surgical knife to take out part or all of an affected area. If lymph nodes are believed to be affected, a biopsy of those will be taken next.

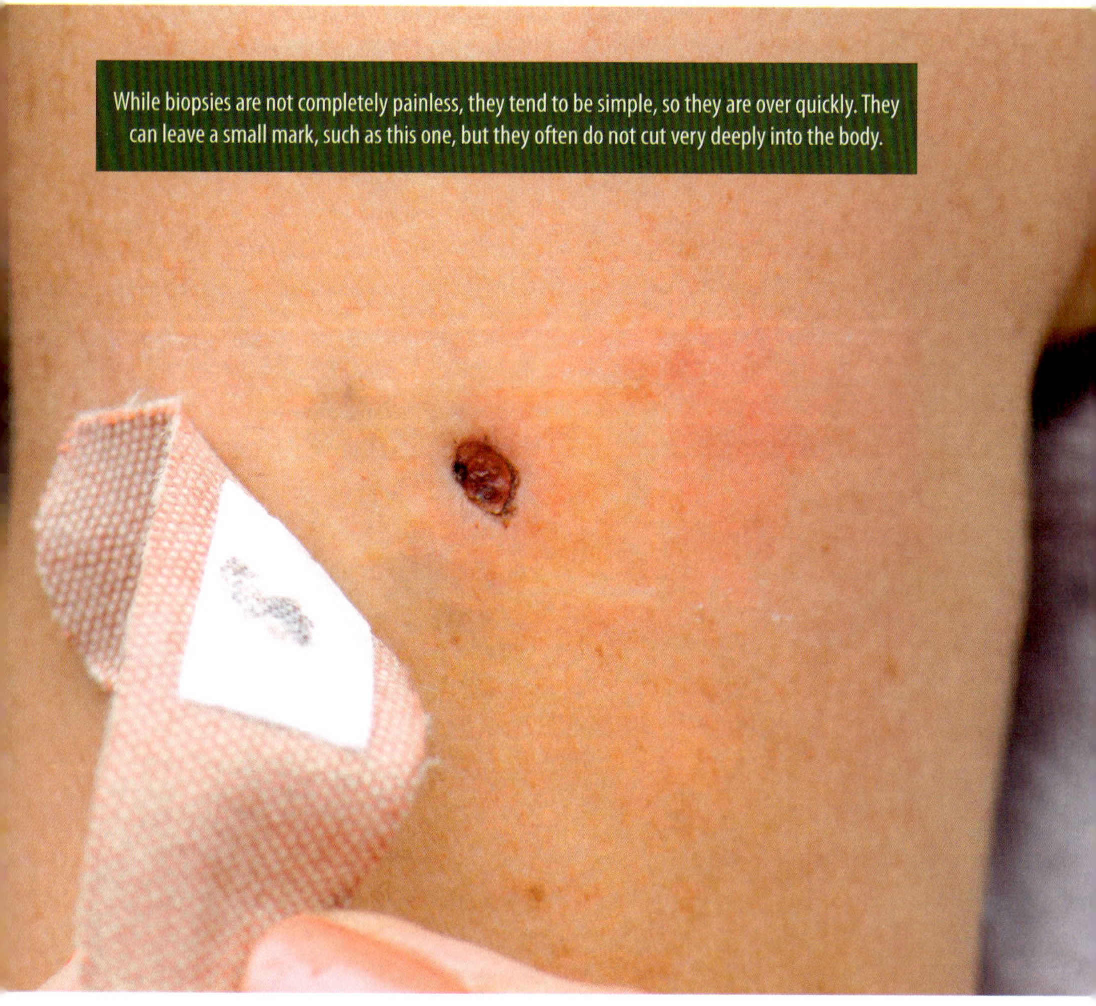

While biopsies are not completely painless, they tend to be simple, so they are over quickly. They can leave a small mark, such as this one, but they often do not cut very deeply into the body.

Lymph node biopsies are often done using a thin needle to remove tissue. The needle is smaller than the needle used for blood tests. In fact, it is so small that the patient may not even need anesthesia. A needle biopsy is used only for large lymph nodes that are near a skin cancer.

The first step in treating skin cancer is to find out what kind of cancer it is. Once a diagnosis is clear, the next step is generally to remove the cancer as quickly as possible. After it is removed, doctors will then focus on preventing the cancer from coming back. They also make sure to monitor the skin with regular checkups, since people who have cancer once have a higher risk of getting it again.

CHAPTER THREE

THE PRECANCER STAGE

Even when it has been sunburned or tanned frequently, skin does not develop cancer overnight. Instead, it changes slowly and gradually, first going through a stage called precancer. The most common type of precancerous growth is called actinic keratosis (AK). This refers to a thick, scaly growth (keratosis, or keratoses if there is more than one) that is caused by sunlight (actinic). Sometimes, actinic keratoses are also referred to as solar keratoses. If left untreated, AK has a chance of developing into squamous cell carcinoma.

Invisible Danger

Although the name means thick and scaly, AKs can be surprisingly hard to spot. They can be as small as an eighth of an inch or grow to a full inch. They are rough, raised, crusty bumps of skin, occasionally horn-like in appearance. They can be pink, red, tan, white, or any combination of those. Sometimes they hide under the surface of the skin where they cannot be seen or felt, and sometimes they disappear and come back later.

AKs can appear on the lips as protruding white, bloody sores. They can also appear on ears, noses, hands, arms, and bald areas on the head. They can appear on any area of skin that has been regularly exposed to sunlight. Unfortunately, they rarely occur alone. Where there is one AK, there are probably more. If only one is visible, the others are generally nearby, lying just under the surface of the skin.

Seeing Similar Patterns

Like skin cancer, AKs are found on people who have spent a lot of time in the sun. Truckers and other people who drive a lot sometimes develop what doctors call "left arm syndrome." Since American drivers sit on the left side of a car, their left forearms and the left sides of their faces are more exposed to sunlight and thus more vulnerable to AKs. People whose jobs take them outside, such as landscapers, construction workers, and some athletes, are also at risk for developing them.

Fair-skinned people are the most likely to develop AKs, especially if they have blonde, red, or thinning hair and blue, green, or grey eyes. Darker-skinned people can also develop AKs if they spend a lot of time in the sun without sunscreen. Furthermore, AK becomes more common as people age. More than 50 percent of men and 33 percent of women who are 65 to 74 years old and have a history of prolonged sun exposure develop them.

Difficult Detection and Recurrence

AKs can be tricky to spot, which is why a dermatologist may use a dermatoscope to find suspected problem areas. When AK is suspected, a biopsy of the skin will answer several questions. Sometimes growths are benign, but others may test as precancerous or cancerous. For example, seborrheic keratoses have rough surfaces, similar to AKs, but these do not develop into cancer. Lipomas are soft growths, but they are formed by ordinary, harmless fat cells. Warts, too, have rough

A Look at Three Other Precancers

AK is the most common type of precancerous skin condition, but it is not the only one. Dermatologists sometimes see three other types of precancer: arsenical keratosis, leukoplakia, and Bowen's disease.

Arsenical keratosis develops in people who have been exposed to arsenic for long periods—for instance, through medications or workplace environments. Like actinic keratosis, arsenical keratosis makes the skin rough, but arsenical keratosis tends to show up on the palms, soles of the feet, and sides of fingers and toes in the form of small, yellow calluses.

Leukoplakia develops as thick white patches on the tongue or inside the mouth. Often, tobacco use is the cause of leukoplakia in the mouth, but it can also be caused by rough edges on dentures and fillings. Leukoplakia is typically painless and benign, but it can lead to more severe issues. Fuzzy white patches in the mouth are sometimes seen in people with weakened immune systems, such as HIV and AIDS patients.

Bowen's disease, named after the doctor who discovered it, shows up as red-brown, scaly patches that can look like psoriasis or eczema, which are two harmless skin conditions. Arsenic; human papillomavirus (HPV), which causes warts; aging; and chronic sun exposure have all been found to cause Bowen's disease. The patches are typically painless but sometimes itchy. They can be removed by a variety of different methods.

All three of these skin conditions are precursors to squamous cell carcinoma, which spreads and grows inward into the layers of the skin. Early detection is the key to preventing further damage or loss of life.

Squamous Cell Carcinoma

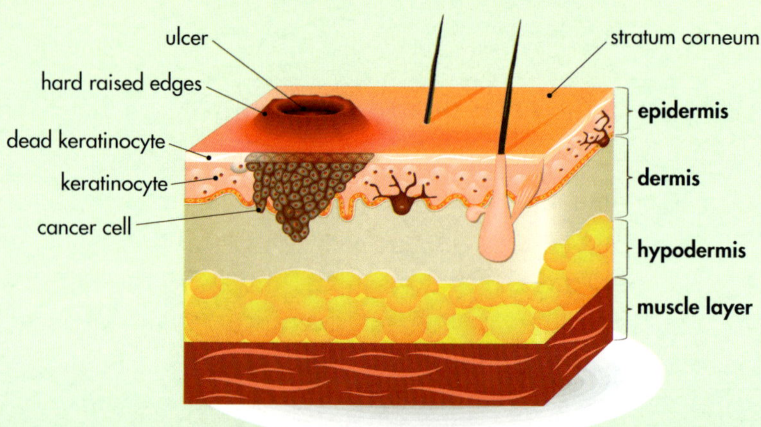

Precancers need to be detected early because they can develop into squamous cell carcinomas. Squamous cell carcinomas are dangerous because they grow into the skin, as shown here. They can spread to other areas of the body as well, making them much more difficult to remove and treat.

surfaces, but those are caused by a virus, not DNA cell damage.

Ordinarily, AKs do not cause any symptoms other than their appearance. They grow very slowly and, for the most part, never develop into cancer. However, some of them do become cancerous, and the chance of this happening is difficult to predict. Left untreated, AKs can develop into squamous cell carcinoma, but AKs are often treated successfully when identified early enough.

Because a patient who gets one AK is likely to get many more, the first part of treatment is frequently education. Dermatologists talk to patients about avoiding further prolonged exposure to the sun and wearing sunscreen every day. They also stress the importance of having regular checkups to find any new AKs that may appear. Many different types of therapies and treatments can then be used.

One Cool Treatment

Cryosurgery dates back about 100 years, and advances in techniques and tools have led to a current 75 to 99 percent success rate with this form of treatment. If a patient has just a few AKs, a dermatologist will often remove them with cryosurgery. Cryosurgery removes growths by freezing them with a spray or swab of liquid nitrogen. The frozen AK will eventually crust and fall off. Although the cryoprobe used in this treatment reaches temperatures of –13°F to –58°F (–25°C to –50°C), it will only damage the tissue it is directly applied to. Dermatologists, therefore, need to be extremely careful not to damage healthy tissue. This procedure can be done as many times as needed. Side effects are minimal, but some discomfort can remain for a little while after cryosurgery.

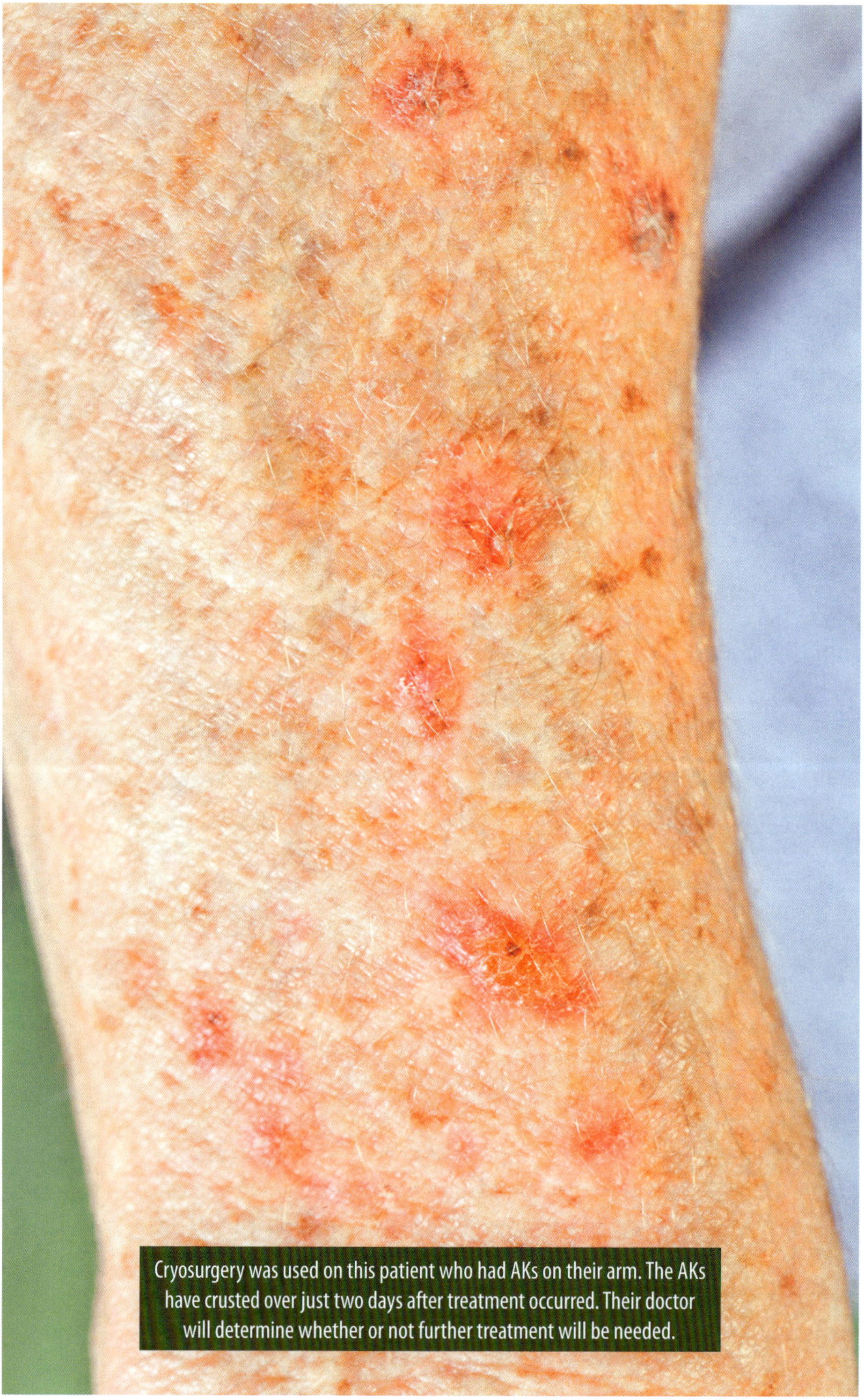

Cryosurgery was used on this patient who had AKs on their arm. The AKs have crusted over just two days after treatment occurred. Their doctor will determine whether or not further treatment will be needed.

Liquid Chemo

When patients have many AKs, dermatologists may prescribe chemotherapy. Unlike the chemotherapy other cancer patients receive intravenously, or through the vein, the chemotherapy used for skin disorders can be applied topically, or on the skin, as a cream. A cream can treat a large area and can reach AKs that are invisible under the surface of the skin.

These creams are incredibly strong and often leave the skin red and sore, but the skin generally clears up within two weeks after the treatment is finished. A small percentage of patients, however, report increased light sensitivity and scarring after treatment.

Making Life More Comfortable

Because many AK treatments can be painful, researchers are looking for more comfortable ways to treat patients. Photodynamic therapy (PDT) is one keratosis treatment that is still being researched to see how it can be improved. PDT uses special drugs called photosensitizing agents, which are placed on the affected skin or into a patient's bloodstream. The chemical solution is eventually absorbed into cancer cells, where a special light is then placed on the cancerous area. This light reacts with oxygen, activating the drug and killing the cancer cells. Although it can be effective, the photosensitizing agent makes skin so sensitive to light that people cannot go outside with their skin uncovered for several days after each round of treatment.

Some studies are looking into PDT to treat deeper problems, such as stomach and brain cancers. Other breakthroughs have been made in improving the photosensitizing drugs that are used, making them faster and more effective. Gels and topical creams are being developed and reformulated to treat AK, with the hope that they will cause less pain for patients.

Dermatologists have also developed some other creams that irritate the skin less than those containing chemotherapy drugs. In 2008, a study was published comparing the effectiveness of a full 5 percent chemotherapy cream to that of a reduced 0.5 percent cream. Not only was the effectiveness found to be the same, but the reduction in medication meant less skin irritation in patients. It was even found to remove AKs more quickly when combined with cryotherapy.

The most typical cream used in this treatment is called 5-fluorouracil (5-FU), and it works by destroying the cancerous cells that are multiplying in the body. However, this also means that some healthy cells are damaged during treatment as well. Scientists, doctors, and researchers are constantly working to develop better and safer treatments.

Under the Knife

When cryosurgery or topical creams are not working as expected, AKs can also be removed with conventional surgery. This is often the case if a doctor is not sure whether the AK has progressed from precancer to cancer. In this case, a biopsy will allow examination of the deeper levels of tissue. Anesthesia is used on the patient undergoing conventional surgery, and any open wound is stitched together after the procedure. Depending on the AK and how deep it is thought to extend into the skin, doctors have several options for surgery.

One option is to excise, or cut out, the whole AK and some nearby tissue, just to make sure it has not spread. Doctors do not choose this option unless they fear that the AK may be developing into cancer.

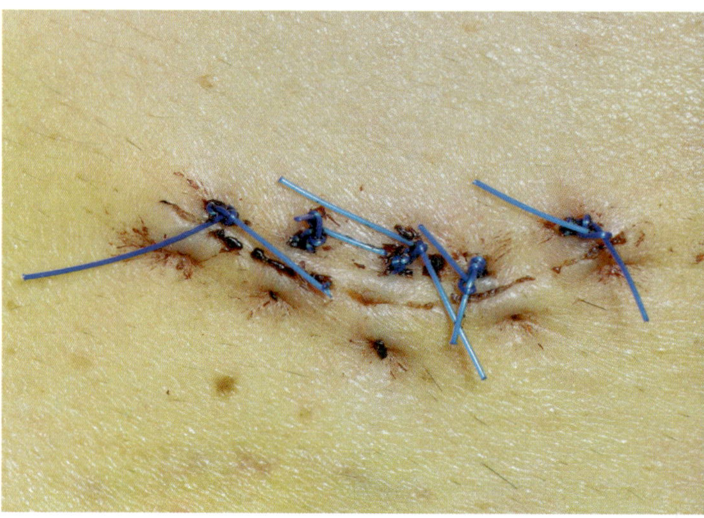

This biopsy required stitching afterward. This kind of procedure often leaves a scar. Protecting the scar from UV exposure is one way to ensure that it heals without becoming too visible.

Another option is to shave off the AK layer by layer, being careful to take only as much tissue as necessary. A third option is to scrape the AK off with a curette (a sharp, spoon-like instrument) and then cauterize the area (burn the wound closed) with electricity. This process is called electrodessication.

A scar will likely remain after conventional surgery. Doctors provide special care instructions for the scar, which typically include limiting the scar's exposure to the sun. UV rays tend to make scars darken and become more visible.

A Controversial Debate

AKs themselves are not fatal, as most never develop into cancer. Many dermatologists believe it is misleading to call them precancerous. To be considered precancerous, skin cells must be abnormal but not malignant. This means they must not yet have spread and invaded other areas of skin. However, if cells have the ability to grow and spread, they are considered precancerous.

AKs are controversial because they seem to fit both definitions. Most AKs never spread, but some do. Because some AKs do develop into cancer if left untreated—about 10 percent, according to the Surgical Dermatology Group—some dermatologists argue that they should be classified as the earliest form of squamous cell carcinoma.

Some researchers believe most AKs would probably develop into cancer if they are left untreated long enough. When AKs do turn into cancer, they become squamous cell carcinomas—one of the two most common forms of skin cancer. Even when AKs themselves do not turn into cancer, a patient has a higher chance of developing skin cancer elsewhere on their body. Patients must seek a doctor upon finding any abnormal skin changes on their bodies.

CHAPTER FOUR

COMMON CARCINOMAS

Basal cell carcinomas and squamous cell carcinomas account for more than 90 percent of all skin cancer cases in the United States. In 2016, the American Cancer Society estimated that "about 5.4 million basal and squamous cell skin cancers are diagnosed each year (occurring in about 3.3 million Americans, as some people have more than one). About 8 out of 10 of these are basal cell cancers. Squamous cell cancers occur less often."[22] Together, these cancers are often referred to as nonmelanoma cancers.

Nonmelanoma cancers are relatively easy to treat, and they tend to be less aggressive than melanomas—and less deadly. While carcinoma cases have been increasing over the years, the death rates have been decreasing. An estimated 2,000 Americans die from nonmelanoma cancers each year, but exact numbers are not known because nonmelanomas are not reported to cancer registries. Patients with weakened immune systems are most likely to die from this type of cancer, as are the elderly. Elderly patients are often too late in having nonmelanomas examined and treated.

One Common Cause

Most people who develop skin cancer have one thing in common: They were exposed to UV radiation from sunlight or from tanning salons. There are three kinds of UV rays, but only two of them cause damage. UVA rays, which are typically used in tanning beds, age skin cells and damage DNA by penetrating the skin deeply. UVB rays are what give people sunburn, causing skin cancer through prolonged periods of exposure. They do not penetrate the skin as deeply as UVA rays. UVA rays play a large role in the creation of melanomas, while UVB rays are more responsible for nonmelanoma cancers. For this reason, people should find a sunscreen that says it blocks both types of rays. The final rays, UVC, do not pass through Earth's atmosphere and therefore do not affect people's skin. Some sunscreens promise to block UVC rays as well, but the Environmental Protection Agency (EPA) and Skin Cancer Foundation both agree that nearly all of these rays are absorbed in the ozone layer of the atmosphere before they reach Earth. As *Refinery29* reported, "With this in mind, Dr. Jeffrey M. Weinberg, a dermatologist at St. Luke's-Roosevelt Hospital Center and Associate Clinical Professor of Dermatology at Mount Sinai School of Medicine, concurs [agrees] that since all UVC should be absorbed by the ozone, any products that claim UVC protection are engaging in marketing hype."[23]

According to the EPA, "Not all melanomas are exclusively sun-related—other possible influences include genetic factors and immune system deficiencies."[24] However, prolonged and chronic sun exposure, as well as a history of sunburn, do increase melanoma and nonmelanoma development.

One reason that basal and squamous cell carcinomas are linked to chronic sun exposure is that they appear in different locations on the body than melanomas do. Melanomas are more common in parts of the body that would be exposed during swimming and sunbathing, such as the legs, the chest, and the back. Basal cell carcinomas, on the other hand, tend to develop on the face, head, and neck.

Squamous cell carcinomas also commonly appear on the head as well. These form in larger masses and easily spread. Basal cell carcinomas can spread as well, but these tend to develop more slowly.

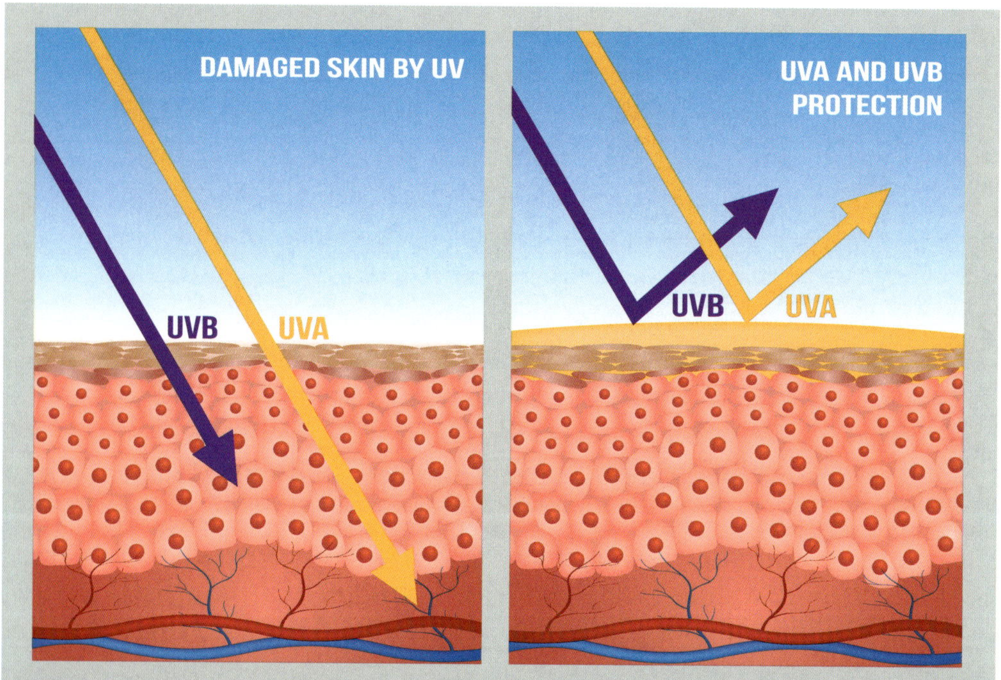

While UVA rays penetrate the skin more deeply than UVB rays, both types of rays can lead to skin cancer if skin is left exposed. The use of broad-spectrum sunscreen will make the majority of these rays reflect right off the skin.

The Limits and Power of Sunscreen

Some people use sunscreen as a way to stay out in the sun longer without getting burned. Dermatologists recommend that people not stay out in the sun for long periods of time, even if they have carefully applied plenty of sunscreen. Research suggests that using sunscreen can reduce the risk of developing AKs, squamous cell carcinomas, and melanomas. However, there is currently no link between sunscreen use and the reduction of basal cell carcinomas. The only way to prevent basal cell carcinomas is to reduce the amount of time skin is exposed to the sun.

Michelle Charlesworth developed a basal cell cancer even though she applied sunscreen regularly. She grew up in the South, swimming and getting a tan every summer. Because of her use of sunscreen, she never had a sunburn. However, when she turned 30, basal cell carcinoma appeared on her cheek. "It's very ironic," she said in an article in *Dermatology Insights*. "The one area of my skin that I thought I was really taking care of was my face. Since age 23, I've worn sunscreen and a hat when I went out in the sun. I don't freckle and I don't have moles. So I didn't fit the average profile of someone that would be prone to skin cancer."[25]

Despite sunscreen's ineffectiveness in preventing basal cell carcinoma, its importance and effectiveness in preventing other skin cancers cannot be understated. Sunscreen should be applied liberally, applied often, and reapplied after excessive sweating or swimming. Furthermore, the FDA has created regulations allowing consumers to easily see if their sunscreen is broad-spectrum. Broad-spectrum sunscreen, which blocks both UVA and UVB rays, provides the best protection.

SPF is the term used for sunscreen, which stands for "sun protection factor." SPF 15 is recommended for everyday regular sun exposure; it will block 93 percent of UVB rays. SPF 30 blocks 97 percent of UVB rays, while SPF 50 blocks 98 percent. Anything above SPF 50 generally does not provide any extra protection. Experts say applying sunscreen correctly and often is more important for protection than a high SPF number.

For those who plan to spend a very long day under the hot sun, the Skin Cancer Foundation recommends using any sunscreen with an SPF of 30 or above.

However, any sunscreen is better than no sunscreen. When used properly, sunscreen will limit the amount of damaging UV rays a person's skin will absorb.

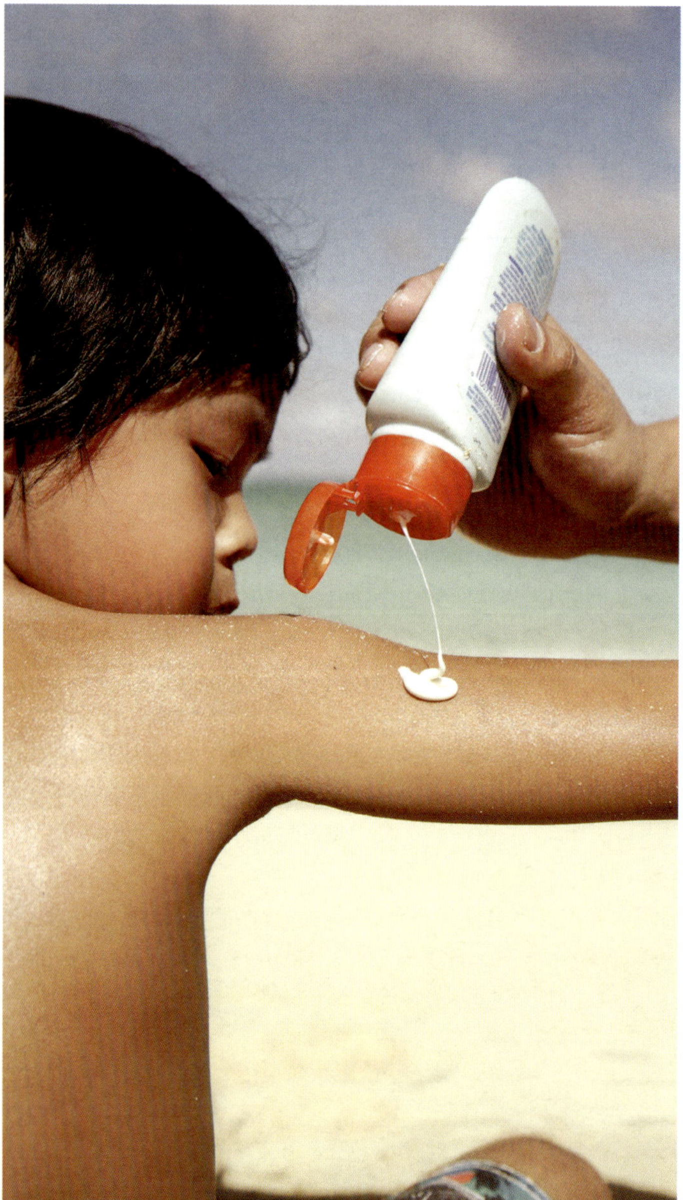

For hard-to-reach places, a helping hand will ensure that sunscreen gets where it needs to be. It should be reapplied every two hours—more often if someone is sweating heavily or goes swimming, even if the sunscreen is labeled as waterproof.

Signs of Basal Cell Carcinoma

In the United States, an estimated 75 percent of skin cancers are basal cell carcinomas. Patients over 60 years of age account for about 90 percent of these basal cell carcinoma cases. Furthermore, the Skin Cancer Foundation has reported that Caucasians, Hispanics, Japanese, and Chinese most commonly develop basal cell carcinoma. This carcinoma is very rare in people with dark skin. Currently, more men than women develop basal cell carcinoma.

The Other 1 Percent

Basal cell carcinoma and squamous cell carcinoma account for 99 percent of nonmelanomas. The other 1 percent can include:

- cutaneous T-cell lymphoma (CTCL): a type of cancer affecting lymphocytes, or white blood cells. These affected blood cells can spread and create tumors in the body. CTCLs appear as itchy, rash-like patches or tumors on the skin. CTCL is treatable, but it is not currently curable. Another form of cutaneous lymphoma, known as cutaneous B-cell lymphoma (CBCL), appears as smoother lumps or rashes.
- Kaposi's sarcoma (KS): brown, red, or purple lesions on the skin or mouth. It becomes life-threatening when these lesions form in the lungs or digestive tract. KS is created by the cells that line blood vessels and lymph nodes. There are different types of this sarcoma, which mainly affect people with HIV, people of African descent, people of Mediterranean descent, and recent recipients of organ transplants.
- Merkel cell carcinoma: painless, red, blue, or purple nodules that form on the head or neck. Recent research has determined that this form of carcinoma is linked to the Merkel cell polyomavirus. Although the virus is commonly found on the skin, this cancer is rare. If left untreated, it spreads quickly to other parts of the body.
- sarcoma: a rare type of cancer that generally develops in the connective tissue deep below the epidermis. There are more than 50 forms of sarcomas that affect soft tissue or bones. Sarcomas can develop anywhere in the body, causing pain as they grow and press up against nerves or muscles. Because sarcomas form inside the body, they are often hard to detect. When found, sarcomas can be removed through surgery.

Basal cell carcinomas tend to grow slowly, but they have a chance of spreading further into the body. They also tend to form in places UV rays touch, especially on the face, eyelids, nose, and the neck. However, it is possible for them to form anywhere. They may look like flat, firm, pale areas of skin. Generally, they are small, raised, pinkish-red, shiny, or waxy bumps. Other times they can appear as pearly white scars or as open sores. The more serious the growth is, the more aggressive treatment needs to be.

Because basal cell carcinomas break open easily, they can appear as cuts or sores on the face or legs. However, because many people shave their faces and legs, they may not think twice about a cut there. Those types of injuries heal within a week or so, unlike basal cell carcinomas, which will not heal at all. They will continue to slowly grow and possibly spread, which is a red flag to get it checked out and treated.

The Second Most Common Skin Cancer

Squamous cells, which make up the uppermost layer of the skin, can be damaged through a lifetime of daily sun exposure or regular visits to tanning salons. UV rays damage the squamous cells and create uncontrollable replication and growth. When this happens, squamous cell carcinoma occurs. It can appear as open sores, warts, or reddish patches of dry skin, and it can lead to disfigurement and sometimes death.

In the past 30 years, squamous cell carcinomas have increased by an estimated 200 percent. More than 1 million cases are diagnosed in the United States every year, with more than 15,000 people dying from it yearly. While it was once most common in people over the age of 50, squamous cell carcinomas are now being diagnosed in people as young as 20. Doctors and researchers attribute the rise of these cases in younger patients to their use of indoor tanning beds. As men tend to spend more time outdoors, they are twice as likely as women to develop squamous cell carcinoma.

Squamous cell cancers can develop anywhere, though they most commonly appear on the ears, lower lip, face, neck, arms, and legs. They become deadly when they spread to organs within the body, and they

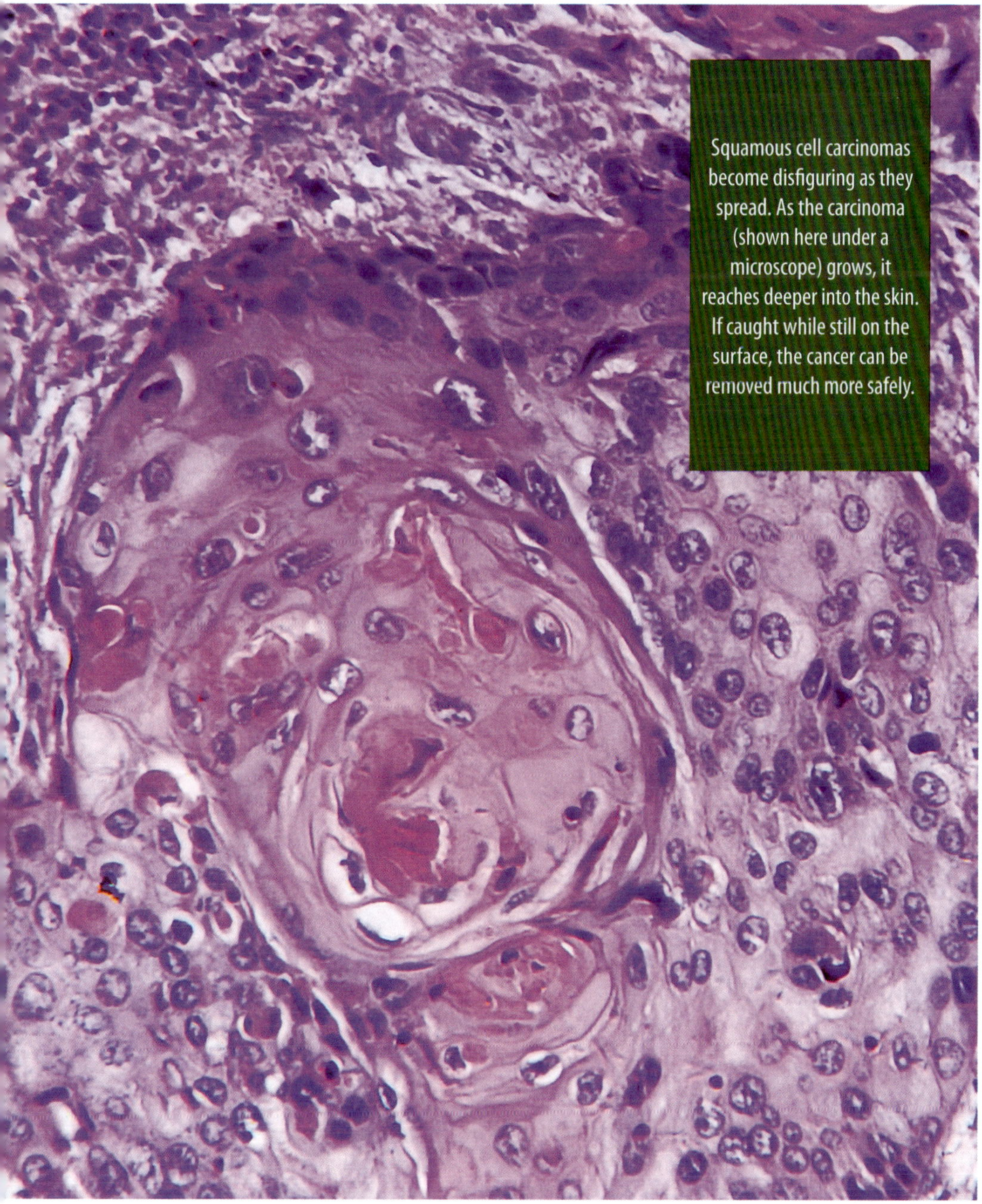

Squamous cell carcinomas become disfiguring as they spread. As the carcinoma (shown here under a microscope) grows, it reaches deeper into the skin. If caught while still on the surface, the cancer can be removed much more safely.

become disfiguring when they affect the other layers of skin tissue. This cancer can also form from ulcers, previous cuts, burns, and even past X-ray exposure. If caught early enough, squamous cell carcinomas can be treated by removing the cancerous tissue. This is highly effective and generally leaves minimal damage.

HPV and Its Link to Cancer

Researchers have discovered that some squamous cell carcinomas may be caused by viruses, not by sun exposure. According to the American Cancer Society, "Most squamous cell anal cancers are linked to infection with the human papillomavirus (HPV), the same virus that causes cervical cancer, as well as many other kinds of cancer."[26] There are more than 100 different strains of HPV, and most of them cause warts; only a few cause cancer. Some strains are transmitted through sexual contact. Others—the ones that cause warts to develop in places such as the hands and feet—are transmitted when someone touches the wart (for instance, by shaking hands with someone who has a wart on their finger) or by touching something the person with the wart touched recently. Dermatologists believe that for HPV to cause cancer, it must be associated with other factors. These factors include things such as smoking, pregnancy, exposure to UV radiation, or suppression of the immune system.

When HPV does cause cancer, it has been associated with skin cancers involving mucous membranes, such as squamous cell carcinoma of the sinuses and the esophagus. HPV can also cause squamous cell carcinomas to develop on the genitals; it is responsible for nearly all cases of cervical cancer, and it also plays a role in penile and anal cancers. The CDC estimates that 30,700 HPV cancers in both men and women develop every year in the United States. Thankfully, about 90 percent of HPV infections go

Understanding the Stages of Cancer

Dermatologists and oncologists (doctors who specialize in cancer) sometimes assign a stage to a cancer. The American Cancer Society describes this staging system as "the process of finding out how much cancer is in a person's body and where it's located. It's how the doctor determines the stage of a person's cancer."[1] Basal cell carcinomas are rarely staged because they so rarely spread. Since squamous cell cancers sometimes spread, they can easily be assigned stages. The staging system allows doctors to predict the general course of a cancer's development. Medical health professionals and hospitals use a widely accepted staging system called the TNM system.

TNM stands for "tumor, nodes, and metastasis." The TNM system is highly in-depth and detailed, and it is updated every six to eight years to include new cancer research developments. After a doctor uses tools such as X-rays and sonograms to see cancer within a patient's body, the letters T, N, and M will then be assigned a coded number or letter. These number and letter codes make it easier to understand the cancer's development. For example, Tis means a tumor is in situ, or on the surface of the skin. A doctor would use that information and determine that they could remove the tumor by surgery. By comparison, T4 means that a tumor is large and has spread deep into tissue. That is much more difficult to treat.

For patients and their families, other versions of the TNM system exist. The most commonly known system is probably the numbered system, in which cancer is assigned one of five numbers. These are typically written as 0, I, II, III, and IV. These numbered stages are all simplified and condensed versions of the much more detailed TNM system. For example, Stage 0 cancer is equal to Tis. Stage IV cancer means the cancer has aggressively spread to other parts of the body. This staging system can be applied to a variety of different cancers and is made to fit a cancer's specific characteristics.

1. "Cancer Staging," American Cancer Society, March 25, 2015. www.cancer.org/treatment/understanding-your-diagnosis/staging.html.

away on their own, and the HPV vaccine prevents an estimated 28,000 infections a year. As with any cancer, screening and early detection are the key in treatment and survival.

The Stages of Squamous Cell Carcinoma

Squamous cell cancers are not very likely to spread to other parts of the body, although they are slightly more likely to spread than basal cell cancers. The Angeles Clinic and Research Institute reported that "some forms of squamous cell carcinoma are aggressive and can spread to other parts of the body, including fat tissues, lymph nodes, and internal organs."[27] Once they do spread to the lymph nodes, they can easily migrate to other parts of the body. A nonmelanoma cancer begins in the earliest stage, which is Stage 0. This is when the carcinoma is in situ, or only on the epidermis.

Stage I and II nonmelanomas are very similar to each other. At these stages, the cancer has hopefully been caught early enough to treat. Stage I and II mean that they have not spread deeply into muscle, cartilage, bone, or the lymph nodes. The difference is that a Stage I cancer is about 0.75 inch (2 cm) or less, while Stage II means that the squamous cell cancer is slightly larger than 2 cm. It can also be applied if a tumor is visibly changing on the surface, making it a higher risk factor.

Stages 0 and I are the most common stages of nonmelanoma skin cancers, while stages III and IV are a bit more rare. Stage III and IV cancers, however, are very serious when they do occur. At Stage III, the cancer has spread below the epidermis. It is invading cartilage, muscle, bones, or one nearby lymph node. It has not, however, spread to organs such as the lungs, liver, or brain. A Stage IV cancer has spread to these organs through the lymphatic system.

If nonmelanoma cancers are detected at Stage II or earlier, they can be easily removed. Someone who has had skin cancer once, however, is at greater risk of getting it again. After having skin cancer once, it is even more important to keep track of changes in one's skin. If cancer does return, there is no guarantee that the next skin cancer will take the same form as the old one. Someone who develops basal cell carcinoma may later develop squamous cell carcinoma or melanoma—or both.

CHAPTER FIVE

RARE, DEADLY, AND STEADY

Melanoma is the rarest of all skin cancers, but it is also the most deadly. Melanomas spread aggressively and can reach almost any other part of the body, including the brain. An estimated 178,000 Americans are expected to have a melanoma diagnosis in 2018 alone. Approximately 91,000 of those cases will be invasive, falling in Stages I, II, III, or IV. The earlier melanoma is detected, the higher the chance of survival is.

Patients diagnosed with Stage I melanoma have about a 97 percent survival rate five years after diagnosis. Those with Stage IV melanoma only have a 15 to 20 percent chance of still being alive after five years. The National Cancer Institute estimated that 9,730 Americans died of melanoma in 2017. The organization reported that in the United States, "rates for new melanoma of the skin cases have been rising on average 1.5% each year over the last 10 years. Death rates have been falling on average 1.2% each year over 2006-2015."[28] From 1982 to 2011, melanoma rates in the U.S. doubled in number. The number of people dying from this type of cancer has been decreasing, but very slowly.

Worldwide, the WHO estimates that more than 65,000 people die from melanoma every year. There is hope that worldwide death rates will eventually fall rather than remain steady. Because these statistics are calculated every five years, new advances in melanoma detection and treatment are not reflected in past numbers. As more advances are made, survival rates should continue to improve, despite the rise in melanoma cases.

Young or Old

People often think of skin cancer as a disease that attacks the middle-aged and elderly. Melanomas, though, do not discriminate by age. While melanoma risks increase as people age, the Melanoma Research Foundation reported, "The incidence of people under 30 developing melanoma is increasing faster than any other demographic group, soaring by 50% in women since 1980."[29] By age 65, the chance of developing melanoma nearly doubles for men. Melanoma also happens to be the second-most diagnosed cancer in people between the ages of 15 and 29, with 500 children being diagnosed every year.

Probability of Developing Melanoma of the Skin

Sex	birth to 49	50 to 59	60 to 69	70 and older
Male	0.5% (1 in 218)	0.5% (1 in 191)	0.9% (1 in 106)	2.6% (1 in 38)
Female	0.7% (1 in 152)	0.4% (1 in 254)	0.5% (1 in 202)	1.0% (1 in 91)

As age increases, a person's risk of developing melanoma generally does, too, as this information from the AIM at Melanoma Foundation shows.

Damaged DNA, Damaged Future

Melanomas are appearing more in young people in part because young skin is especially sensitive to UV radiation. The average person could potentially double their risk of melanoma with one blistering sunburn. In a 20-year study by the American Association for Cancer Research, researchers "found that those who had at least five blistering sunburns when they were 15 to 20 years old had a 68 percent increased risk for basal cell carcinoma (BCC) and squamous cell carcinoma (SCC) of the skin, and an 80 percent increased risk for melanoma."[30]

In babies and children, there is also a strong link between childhood sunburn and future melanoma development. Children are too young to have developed all of their melanin, so they have less sun protection than adults. Although sunburns increase a person's risk of melanoma, regular, chronic sun exposure does not. In fact, according to the AIM at Melanoma Foundation, "Intermittent exposure to intense sunlight is more strongly associated with the development of melanoma than continuous daily sun exposure."[31]

For example, this means that a person is more likely to develop melanoma if they stay inside on weekdays but spend weekends and vacations in the sun. It is important to note that any UV exposure, whether through sunlight or tanning salons, increases the future risk of developing melanoma. Women between the ages of 16 and 49 are especially drawn to tanning salons, despite the evidence about its risks. It is estimated that tanning before the age of 35 will increase a person's chance of developing melanoma later in life by 75 percent.

Because society associates tanned skin with beauty and health, many people choose to get a tan—either from the sun or a tanning bed—despite the risks. However, beauty products called self-tanners are available that give people a tanned look without exposing them to UV rays. They come in many forms, including creams, sprays, towelettes, and gels. Guidelines to help people choose the best product for their individual needs and tips for the best ways to apply it can be found online. Dermatologists recommend using self-tanners instead of going tanning.

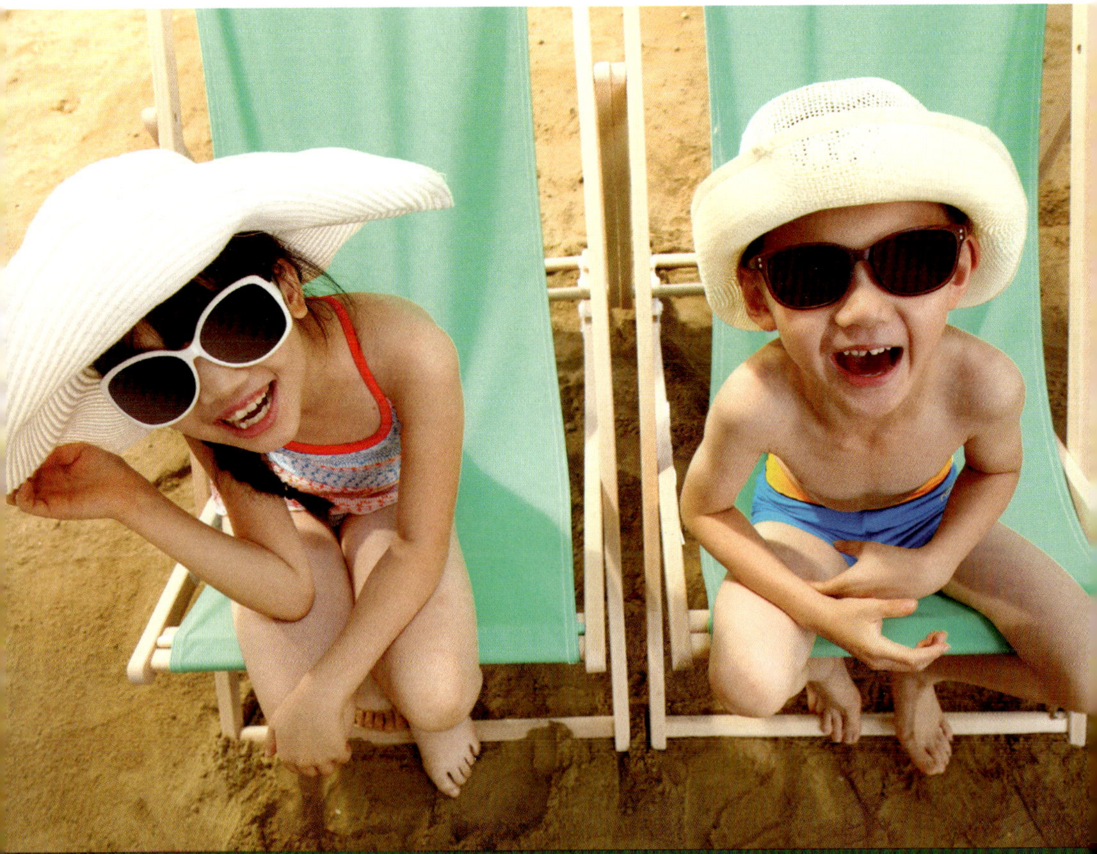

Because childhood sunburn is linked to melanoma in the future, it is important for parents to protect their children from the sun. Sunscreen and a wide-brimmed hat are perfect for a sunny day at any age, but especially for young people. A dark shirt would provide extra protection.

The History of You

Family history can also increase a person's risk of developing melanoma. People who have family members with dysplastic nevi—groups of abnormal moles—have a much higher risk of developing melanoma. In fact, dysplastic nevi increase this risk by an estimated 10 to 12 percent, compared to those who do not have them. Having a close relative who has had melanoma also greatly increases a person's risk, as does the number of moles a person has. The Skin Cancer Foundation recommends that those with a higher risk use sun protection often and perform skin examinations every month, both by themselves and with a professional.

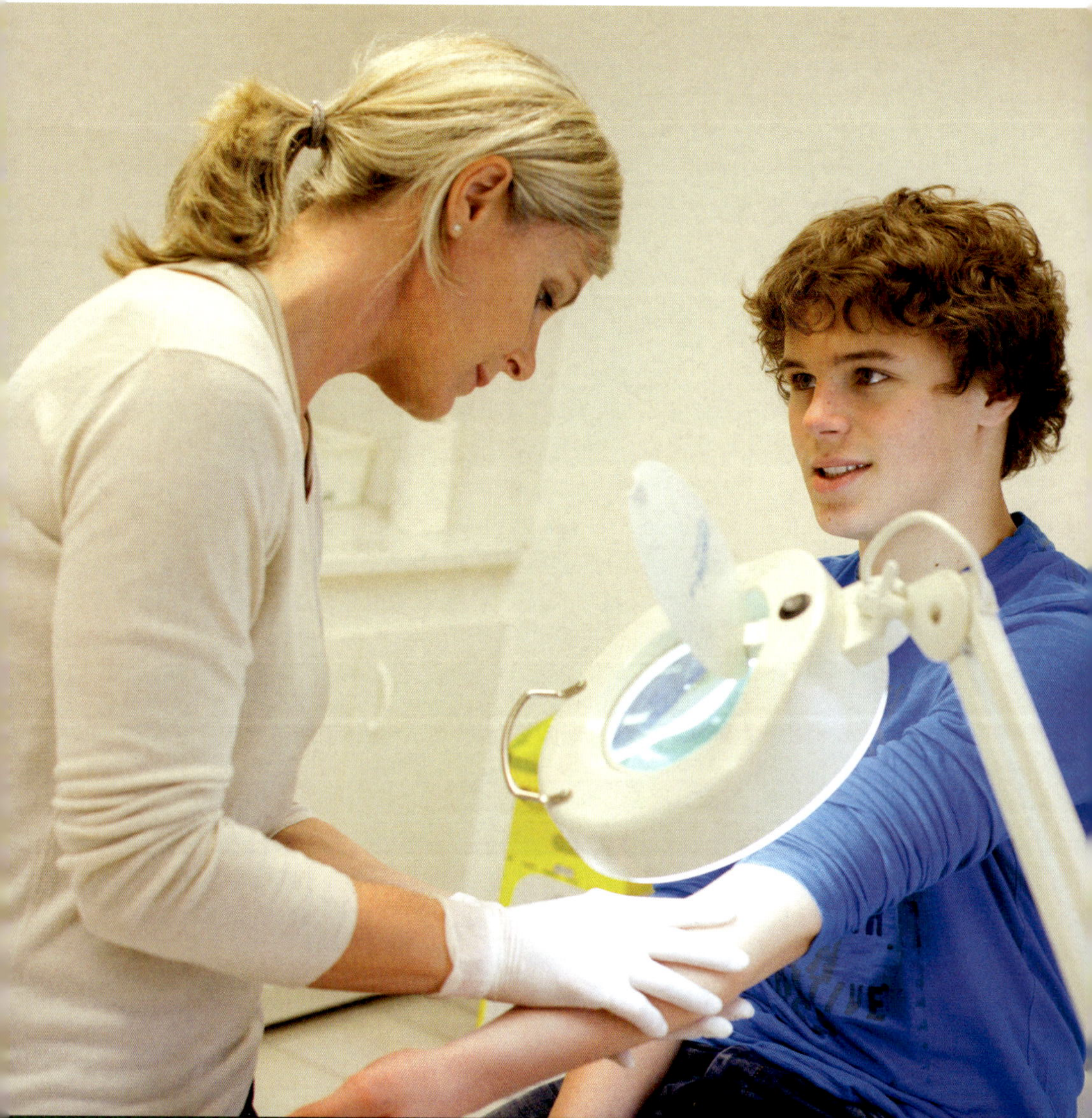

For a person with many moles, a skin screening with a dermatologist is one of the first steps in detecting and identifying melanoma early. If the moles are found to be abnormal or if the patient has a close relative with similar moles, the risk of developing melanoma greatly increases.

Ethnicity, Gender, and Melanoma

As reported by the AIM at Melanoma Foundation, "Caucasian-Americans are 26 times more likely to develop melanoma than African-Americans."[32] Data from the CDC in 2014 backed up this statement. The CDC reported that Caucasian, or white, men were the most likely to develop melanoma, followed by Native American and Asian men. African American men were least likely to develop melanoma. Between 1999 and 2014, the incidence of melanoma cases increased by about 9 percent for men of all races.

During that same time period, the patterns for women were similar, with Caucasian women having the highest melanoma rates and African American women having the lowest. Latinx women were slightly more likely to develop melanoma compared to Native American women, which was the opposite of the male racial trend. However, like the men, women's melanoma rate increased by about 9 percent. Death rates from melanoma showed similar patterns for both genders, with Caucasian men and women being more likely to die from it, followed by Latinx and African Americans.

Melanoma Biopsies

If a visual exam makes a doctor think that a mole might be a melanoma, they can take a sample of the skin to examine more closely under a microscope. When a dermatologist suspects a nonmelanoma cancer, they might choose to biopsy the skin by shaving off a layer at a time and looking at the layers under a microscope. However, when melanoma is suspected, doctors feel it is generally safer to do an excisional biopsy, taking out the entire mole with a surgical knife because of how quickly it can spread.

If a melanoma has metastasized, or spread, doctors sometimes need to do additional testing to find out how far it has spread. One option is to check the lymph nodes near the affected area by doing a needle biopsy. If a needle biopsy does not find any melanoma cells, but the lymph node is still swelling in ways that make doctors suspect that the melanoma has spread, it may be necessary to surgically remove the lymph node.

From Ancient Egypt to Today

It is not unusual for skin cancer patients to be disfigured by their disease. Skin cancer is common on the face and head, so some patients may lose their eyes, ears, or nose. It makes most people feel self-conscious if others stare at them because they are missing parts of their body. These patients, though, can choose to have plastic surgery to reconstruct a damaged body part. As technology improves, so does the prosthetic process.

The use of prosthetics is an ancient process that dates back to the ancient Egyptians, when replacement body parts were made out of silver, gold, clay, or wood. Today, however, tinted silicone is used for creating artificial noses, which are specifically designed to fit a patient's face. This is done by taking a mold of a patient's face and designing a prosthetic that perfectly fits a damaged area.

A rhinectomy (surgery to replace the nose with a prosthetic) is a common option for skin cancer patients who have suffered from carcinoma or melanoma on their noses. Once the carcinoma or melanoma is removed, the nose may be left severely disfigured. The prostheses are made by anaplastologists. These doctors can construct the body parts by mixing small amounts of color with silicone. They even add age-appropriate wrinkles and veins, making prosthetics look so good that most people think they are real.

Some of these man-made replacement parts are external, while others are internal prosthetic implants. This means that some prosthetics are held on by adhesives or magnets, while others can be more securely attached and anchored to bones. In the past, patients were embarrassed by prosthetic noses or ears that were not attached well and could fall off. Internal implants are changing this once common problem by making prosthetics more permanent.

Stages and Survival

As with other cancers, doctors assign a stage to each melanoma they diagnose. The stage indicates whether a melanoma has spread and how much. A patient's prognosis, or chance of recovery, depends on the stage of the melanoma.

If a melanoma is caught in Stage 0 or I, the prognosis is great. Stage 0 is in situ, while Stage I has reached into the next layer of skin. By Stage II, the melanoma is thicker and has a much higher chance of spreading, but the prognosis is still good.

Stage III melanomas have spread deeper into nearby skin or lymph nodes but have not traveled to other parts of the body. The five-year rate of survival for patients in Stage III is about 62 percent. Once the melanoma has reached the lymph nodes, however, it is able to travel to other organs and becomes much harder to treat. This happens in Stage IV melanoma. The brain, bones, and lungs are the most common sites of spreading.

Imaging Scans and Tests

If doctors suspect a melanoma has spread but they are not sure what organs or lymph nodes it may have spread to, a patient may need to have imaging tests done. There are a number of different scans a doctor can perform, which include chest X-rays, CT (or CAT) scans, MRIs, PET scans, and even a specific blood test. These tests can also be used to determine how well cancer treatment is going and to see whether cancer has recurred.

- Chest X-rays are used to see if melanoma has spread to the lungs.
- A computerized tomography (CT) or computerized axial tomography (CAT) scan takes detailed cross-sectional X-rays to look for enlarged lymph nodes or spots on the lungs or liver, all of which are signs of spreading melanoma.
- Magnetic resonance imaging (MRI) uses strong magnets and radio waves to produce cross-sectional images. MRIs are used to look at the brain and spinal cord.

- In a positron emission tomography (PET) scan, radioactive glucose molecules are injected into the body, where they appear in cancer cells. Cancer cells absorb more glucose than ordinary cells do.
- As melanoma spreads, lactate dehydrogenase (or LDH) will appear in higher levels in the blood, so an LDH blood test can indicate whether the levels are high enough to cause concern.

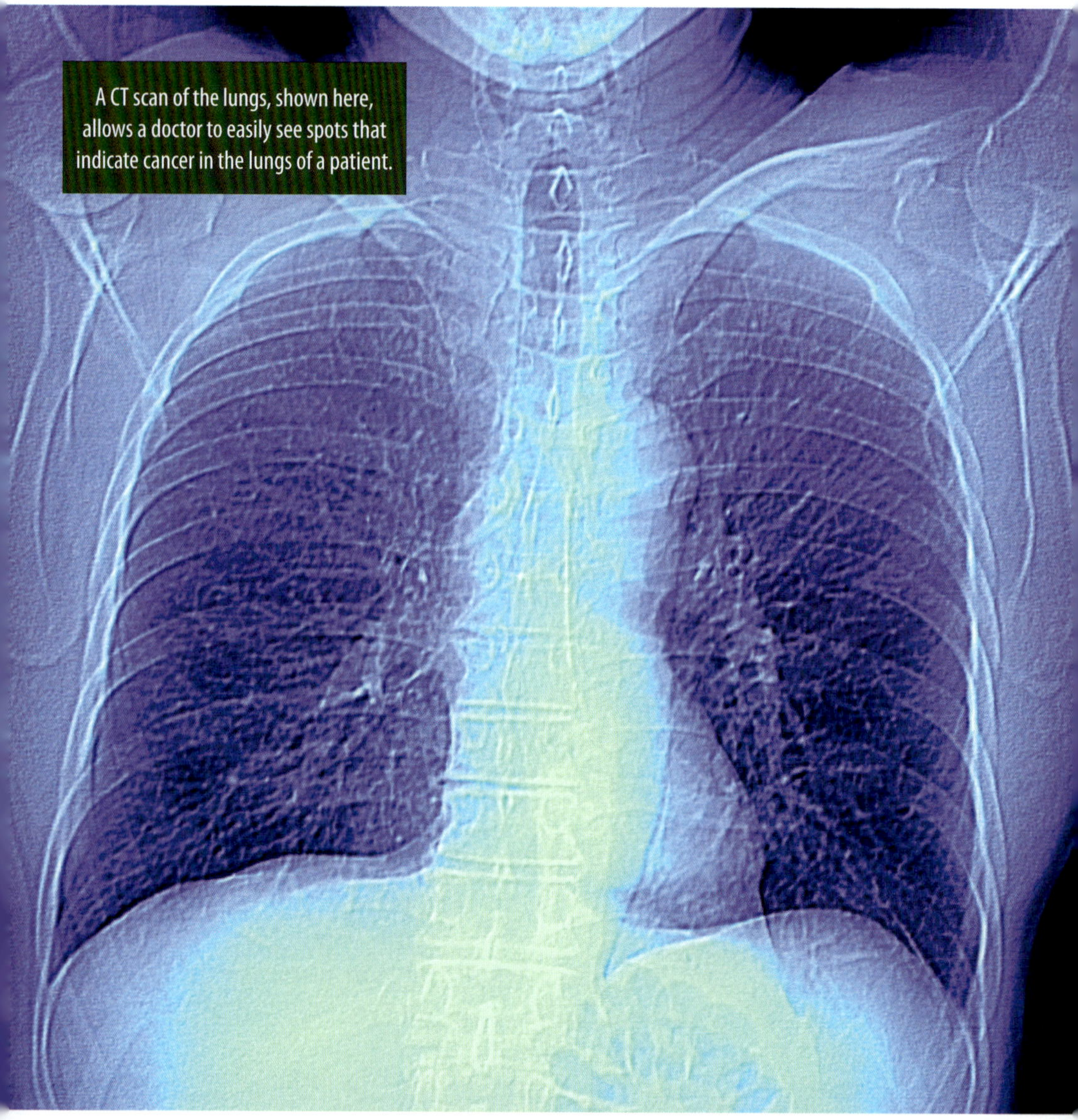

A CT scan of the lungs, shown here, allows a doctor to easily see spots that indicate cancer in the lungs of a patient.

Surviving Melanoma

Melanoma, like any skin cancer, can be difficult to fight and scary to live with. Melanoma, however, is treatable and survivable, although it is often a difficult fight. Melanoma survivor Jamie Troil Goldfarb explained how a battle with cancer can shift a person's perspective on life:

> *We don't sit passively by while cancer happens to us, surviving each day by luck. We fight as hard as we possibly can. We endure levels of physical and emotional pain that most people cannot imagine. We kick, punch, and claw our way out of melanoma's grasp. We don't merely survive it, we conquer it. We are victors. And as victors, we wrestle and steal every ounce of love, gratitude, and beauty out of our journeys. We keep it safe and deep within us, and use it to remind ourselves of just how beautiful life is and how lucky we are to be living it. Because of our victories, we celebrate the mundane, we see joy in the ordinary, and we give thanks for monotonous [boring] every-day routines.*[33]

CHAPTER SIX

TREATING SKIN CANCER

The treatment for skin cancer always depends on how far the cancer has progressed. A cancer that has been detected at a very early stage can often simply be removed. Cancers that have spread, however, may require a whole area of the body, or even the whole body, to be treated. Patients and their doctors must also consider what type of skin cancer they are dealing with and where it is located.

No treatment is perfect; surgeries can leave scars, for instance, and the strong chemicals needed to kill cancerous cells can cause equally strong side effects, such as nausea and irritation of the skin. Additionally, not all treatments are effective, especially if the cancer has spread. However, researchers are constantly looking for new and improved techniques to kill cancerous cells with as few side effects as possible.

Various Surgical Options

Treatment for skin cancer generally begins with surgery. The top layer of the skin, the epidermis, does not contain blood vessels or lymphatic vessels that could transport cancer cells to other parts of the body. Therefore, if a cancer is very small and thin and is confined to the epidermis, removing just this layer of skin may be enough to treat it.

One surgical option is to take the entire cancer out, along with a safety margin of skin around it to make sure every single cancer cell has been removed. If even one remains, it can continue growing and spreading. This method is called simple excision, which is similar to an excisional biopsy. The difference between the two is that a simple excision will remove more of the normal, healthy skin than a biopsy will. The doctor will remove the lesion and surrounding skin in an elliptical (football) shape. This shape allows the area to be stitched, leaving a small scar when it heals.

If a patient has already had a biopsy that removed the cancer and the diagnosis was basal or squamous cell carcinoma, it may not be necessary to do more surgery. However, if the diagnosis was melanoma, the surgeon may feel that it is safer to go back and remove more skin. That way, the remaining skin can be examined to be sure that no cancer cells remain. This is called a re-excision.

In melanoma cases, if the cancer is on a finger or toe, sometimes the cancer is treated with amputation, which means cutting off the entire finger or toe. Years ago, doctors also used to amputate arms and legs to prevent the spread of melanoma, but advances in medical techniques mean that amputations are rare. Surgeons may also remove the lymph nodes, but only if they are enlarged and a lymph node biopsy shows that they contain cancer cells.

Mohs Micrographic Surgery

If a person's skin cancer is on their face, they may be concerned about being disfigured by surgery. Surgeons try to minimize scarring and disfigurement on the face by using the Mohs technique, where a surgeon removes skin one layer at a time with a scalpel and checks the skin immediately under a microscope. If it contains malignant cancer cells, the surgeon removes another layer and checks it. This process continues until a cancer-free layer is reached. Mohs surgery

Circadian Clocks and Cancer Cells

Most living organisms on Earth have an internal clock, known as a circadian rhythm, within their bodies. A person's circadian rhythm regulates biological functions in the body. For instance, it determines what time people start to feel sleepy or when their cells need to divide. When cell division is working properly, it leads to things such as the creation of new skin cells to heal a cut; when it is not working, it leads to the development of tumors. The circadian rhythm also affects the body's response to DNA damage in the body, which typically occurs after UV ray exposure.

In a January 2018 study, researchers from three universities reported that specific hormone receptors that control elements of this circadian rhythm were actually effective in killing cancer cells. The study was performed on mice, two of which exhibited signs of brain cancer. Because cancer cells depend on cell division and metabolism to grow and spread, the researchers targeted specific hormones in the circadian rhythm that control those functions.

The study also set out to block specific pathways in cancer cells by blocking fat and nutrient development, both of which are required for duplication. Precancerous cells in mice were observed to stop growing after this treatment, and the two mice with brain cancer were observed to have a longer lifespan and reduced size in tumors. Scientists and researchers are very optimistic about what the future holds for these findings and how they can be applied to humans.

There is still plenty of research and testing that needs to be done before anything can be tested on humans. As the National Cancer Institute explained, "Scientists are developing drugs that activate or repress other circadian clock components ... and it is possible that combinations of different clock-targeting drugs or of clock-targeting drugs with other types of therapy might enhance anticancer effects. But, currently, there are more questions than there are answers."[1]

1. "New Cancer Treatment Approach Targets Circadian Clock," National Cancer Institute, February 13, 2018. www.cancer.gov/news-events/cancer-currents-blog/2018/targeting-circadian-clock-cancer.

allows surgeons to remove the smallest amount of skin possible.

The entire procedure can last for several hours, but it tends to be a minor surgery. Doctors take great care to keep track of where the skin is being taken from by using a special map. Patients should expect to wait long periods of time as their skin samples are tested in a laboratory. Depending on how intensive the procedure ends up being, doctors might recommend plastic surgery for areas that will not heal smoothly on their own. Plastic surgery, if required, can reconstruct parts of noses or ears to give patients a better quality of life.

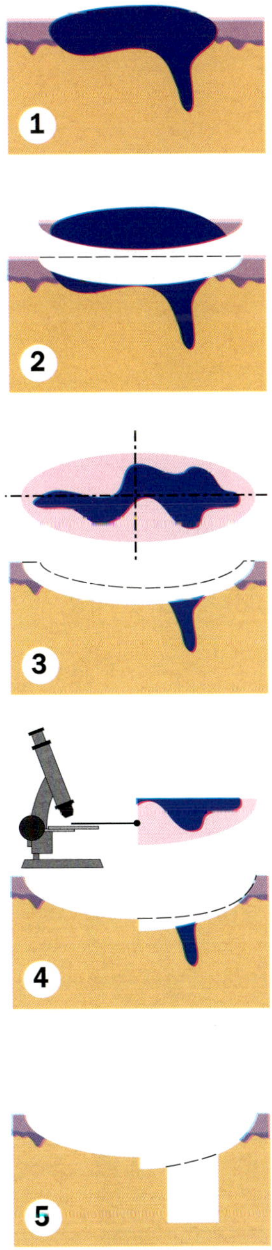

This diagram illustrates how the Mohs technique is designed to minimize skin damage. Layer by layer, skin is removed until a cancer-free layer is reached. This technique ensures that only the cancerous tissue is removed, avoiding as much healthy tissue as possible.

Three Other Techniques

Melanomas are generally treated with simple excision or with Mohs surgery. However, doctors have other options for working with basal and squamous cell carcinomas. One option is for the surgeon to remove the lesion using a curette, which is a sharp, spoon-like instrument. After the lesion is gently scraped off with the curette, the area is treated with an electrical current, administered through a small needle, to cauterize it (stop the bleeding) and kill any remaining cancer cells. This technique is called electrodessication and curettage, and it is effective about 95 percent of the time.

Smaller lesions are sometimes removed with cryosurgery. This technique is often used to remove AKs, but it can also be used for nonmelanoma cancers. A doctor freezes the lesion by applying liquid nitrogen, and over a period of several weeks, the tissue that was frozen dies and falls off. Compared to curettage and electrodessication, the cure rate for cryosurgery is smaller at only about 90 percent.

Laser beam treatment is still being researched and tested, although it is not currently FDA approved. Using a high-intensity beam, laser surgery can be used to destroy and reduce lesions as well as reduce bleeding as it cauterizes blood vessels. Scarring with this type of procedure is high, but it allows doctors more precision in removing cancerous layers of skin.

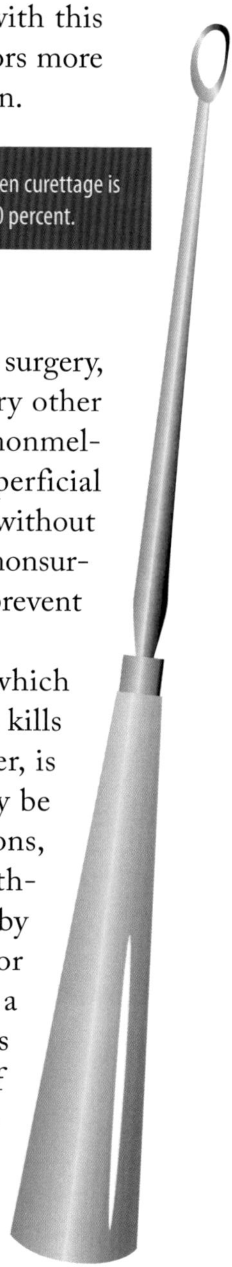

Curettes such as this one are important tools in removing cancerous tissue. When curettage is combined with electrodessication, cure rates are very high—close to 100 percent.

Surgery Not Required

Some patients' bodies are too weak to tolerate surgery, and some people get nervous and want to try other methods first if possible. If someone has a nonmelanoma cancer that is small enough and superficial enough that doctors feel they can be treated without surgery, other approaches can be used. These nonsurgical treatments can also be used as a way to prevent cancer from coming back.

Radiation is one nonsurgical approach, which often focuses on a specific area of skin and kills abnormal cells there. This method, however, is not very precise, so some healthy tissue may be affected as well. For more precise applications, it is possible to irradiate a cancer from within through internal radiation. This is done by inserting radioactive needles, seeds, wires, or pellets inside or near the cancer through a small tube called a catheter. These implants contain either a high dose or low dose of radioactivity. High-dose therapy uses these implants for only minutes at a time, whereas low-dose therapy allows for the implants to remain in the body permanently. The

Melanoma Treatment Today and Tomorrow

Researchers, scientists, and doctors are constantly working to improve cancer detection and treatment techniques. Melanoma treatment is no exception, with the Food and Drug Administration (FDA) approving new medicines and treatments every year. According to the American Cancer Society, new drugs and treatments that have been developed in recent years are actually performing better than traditional chemotherapy treatment. These include:

- radiation therapy: This uses a strong, high-energy, external beam (the way an X-ray does) to destroy cancerous cells. The area of the body where this beam is targeted tends to experience some discomfort, often creating painful skin or, in some cases, fluid buildup. Topical creams help reduce discomfort, as do changes in how the beam is targeted and applied.
- immunotherapy: This therapy aims to build up a body's defenses to fight cancer, by using natural or lab-created substances. These substances can include things such as proteins, inhibitors, or even antibodies, as seen in some cancer vaccines. In October 2015, the FDA approved a treatment that decreases melanoma recurrence, but with severe side effects. In 2017, the FDA approved another immunotherapy drug for Stage III melanoma.
- lymphatic mapping: This technique involves injecting a substance that attaches to cancer cells—along with a blue dye to make it visible—into lymph nodes to see which nodes the substance travels to. Any node that takes in the dye is checked for melanoma cells. If those cells are present, then the affected nodes can be removed through lymph node dissection.
- lymph node dissection: While currently accepted and performed by doctors, studies and tests are being carried out to determine its true effectiveness in improving melanoma survival rates. Depending on how far the tumor has spread, either some or all of the lymph nodes from that area may be removed to try to stop the spread of melanoma.

None of these treatments are 100 percent effective, nor are they always 100 percent safe. However, science, research, and medicine continue to help make advances and save lives.

low-dose implants naturally lose their radioactive properties over time, so people do not have to worry about long-term harm.

Another option is chemotherapy, which uses drugs to stop cancer cells from growing. The drugs may kill the cancer cells or simply stop them from reproducing. If a cancer is a very superficial nonmelanoma, a dermatologist may prescribe a chemotherapy cream that can be applied topically. If the cancer has spread to other parts of the body, though, it may be necessary to treat the whole body with chemotherapy. In that case, chemotherapy drugs are taken by mouth or intravenously. Then, the drugs travel through the bloodstream and attack cancer cells throughout the body in the lymph nodes and organs. Side effects such as hair loss and nausea tend to stop after treatment ends.

Some skin cancer patients are prescribed immunotherapy drugs. These drugs work differently from chemotherapy. Chemotherapy works by attacking cancer cells directly, whereas immunotherapy drugs work by stimulating the body's immune response. Several types of

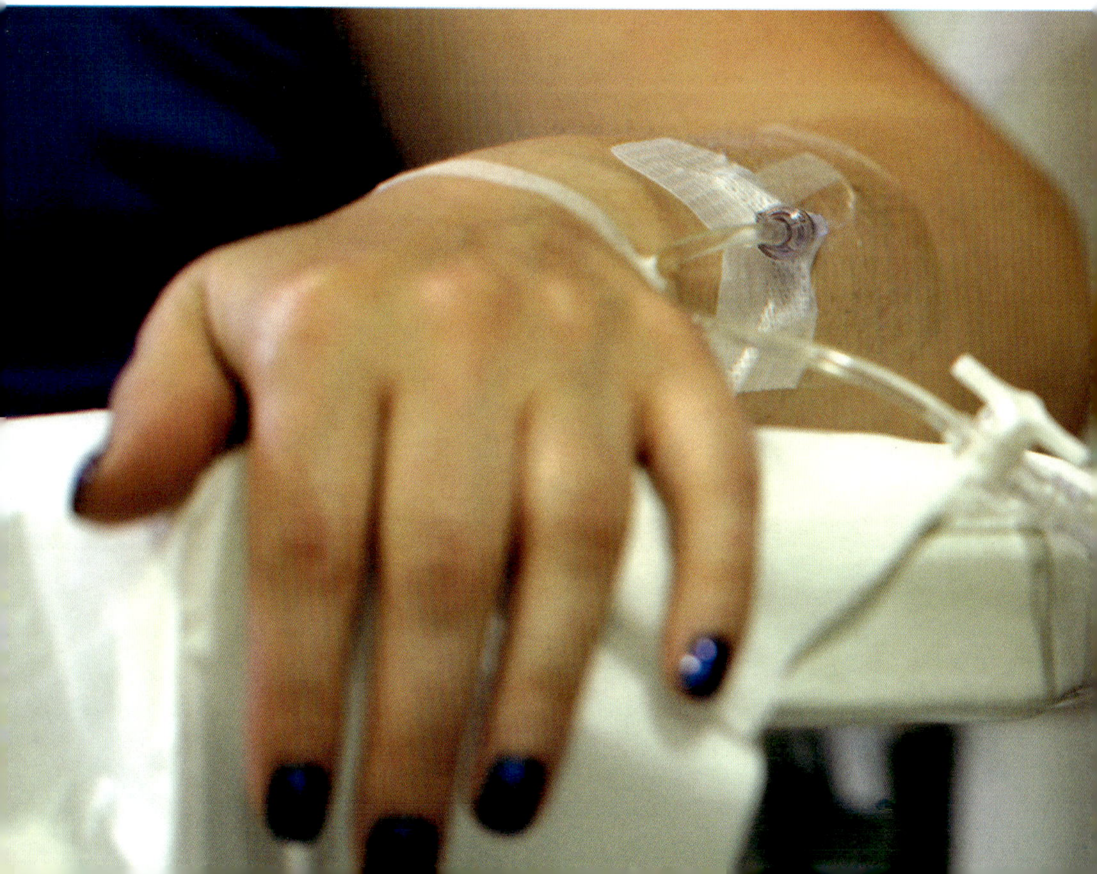

immunotherapy exist, but they all work generally the same way: by using inhibitors to boost immune system protein cells. These inhibitors are given to patients intravenously. The body's own immune system can then kill the cancer cells or stop them from reproducing. One immunotherapy drug can also be applied as a cream.

Doctors can also use photodynamic therapy. This approach involves applying special photosensitizing drugs either on the skin or in the blood. The drugs are eventually absorbed by cancer cells, and a light is then applied to the area where the cancer is. This light reacts with oxygen, creating a chemical that will kill the cancer cells. This therapy, however, only works if light can be applied to the area, so it cannot be used for cancer that has spread to internal organs. Newer phototherapy treatments are being tested to make the drugs faster and more selective against cancer cells.

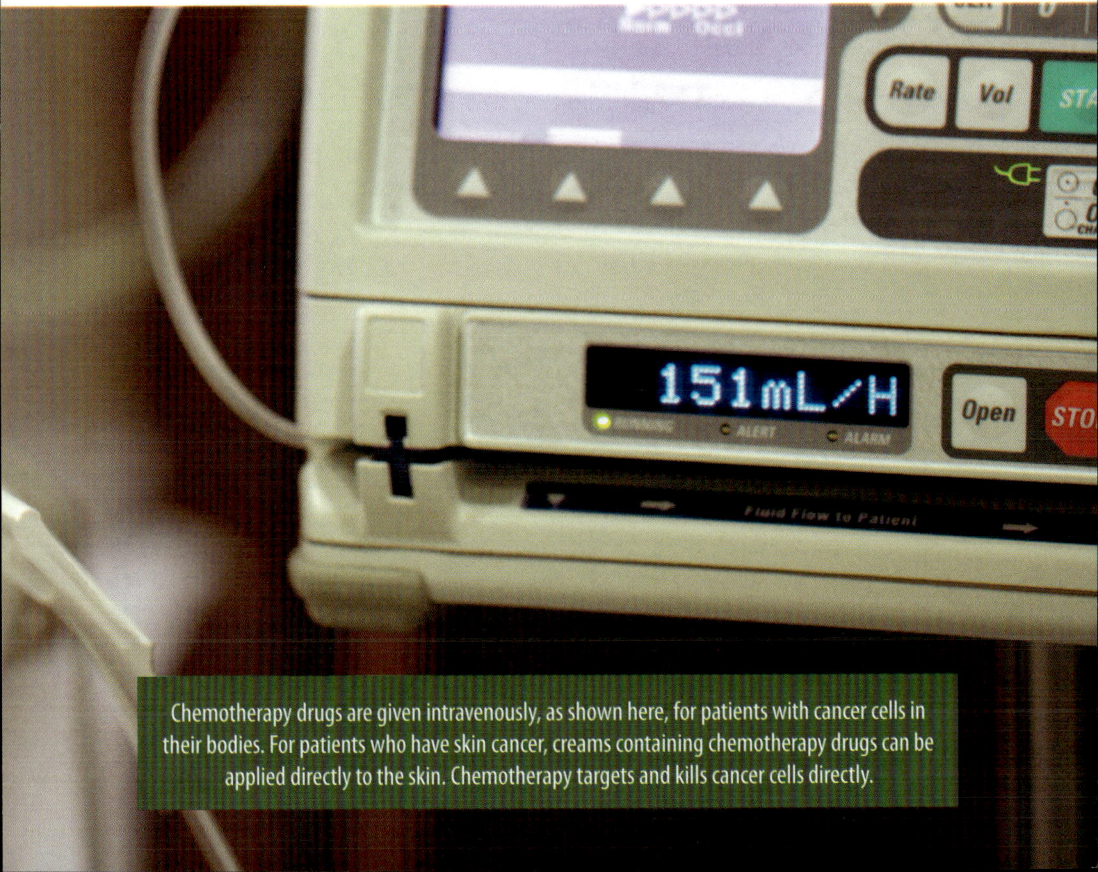

Chemotherapy drugs are given intravenously, as shown here, for patients with cancer cells in their bodies. For patients who have skin cancer, creams containing chemotherapy drugs can be applied directly to the skin. Chemotherapy targets and kills cancer cells directly.

CAM and Integrative Medicine

Some cancer patients are not satisfied with the options presented to them by medical doctors. They choose to supplement their care with complementary medicine, which is when a patient uses non-mainstream techniques or regimens along with ordinary medical care—for instance, taking vitamins or herbs. In alternative medicine, these techniques or regimens are used in place of standard medical care. Complementary and alternative medicine for cancer is collectively referred to as CAM. A fourth practice, known as integrative medicine, combines standard medical care and CAM treatments under a doctor's supervision. Integrative medicine is intended to address all aspects of a patient's treatment—the mind, the body, and the spirit.

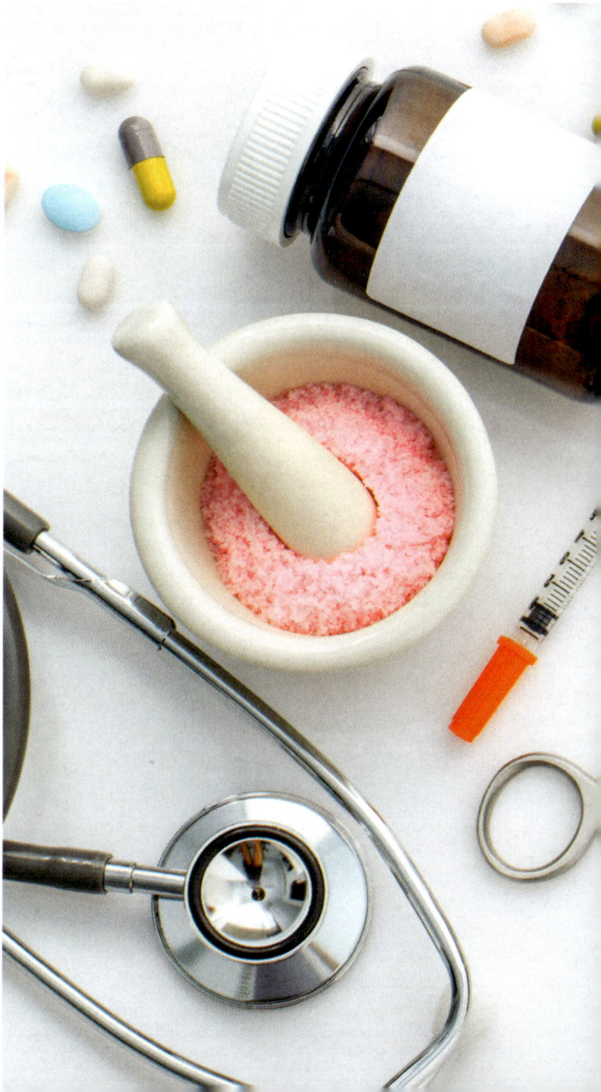

Integrative medicine uses elements of CAM that have been proven and tested to be effective and safe, but not all CAM treatments are tested as rigorously as FDA-approved ones. Some people believe treatments that can be found in nature, such as herbs, are safer than those that are made from chemicals in a laboratory, such as chemotherapy drugs. However, the truth is that some "natural" remedies and dietary supplements may be harmful in large doses or when combined with certain medicines and many are not as effective alone as when combined with standard medical treatments. For this reason, discussions with a doctor before using CAM treatments are very important. The National Center for Complementary and Integrative Health, the NCI Office of Cancer Complementary and Alternative Medicine, and the Office of Dietary Supplements are all government-related organizations that provide factual research on the validity, safety, and effectiveness of various natural and alternative medicines.

The use of all-natural remedies over traditional medicine is tempting for some, despite the lack of FDA approval. While some natural remedies may be harmless, others are sold completely untested and unregulated. Some natural ingredients may also cause a negative reaction when combined with FDA-approved cancer treatments.

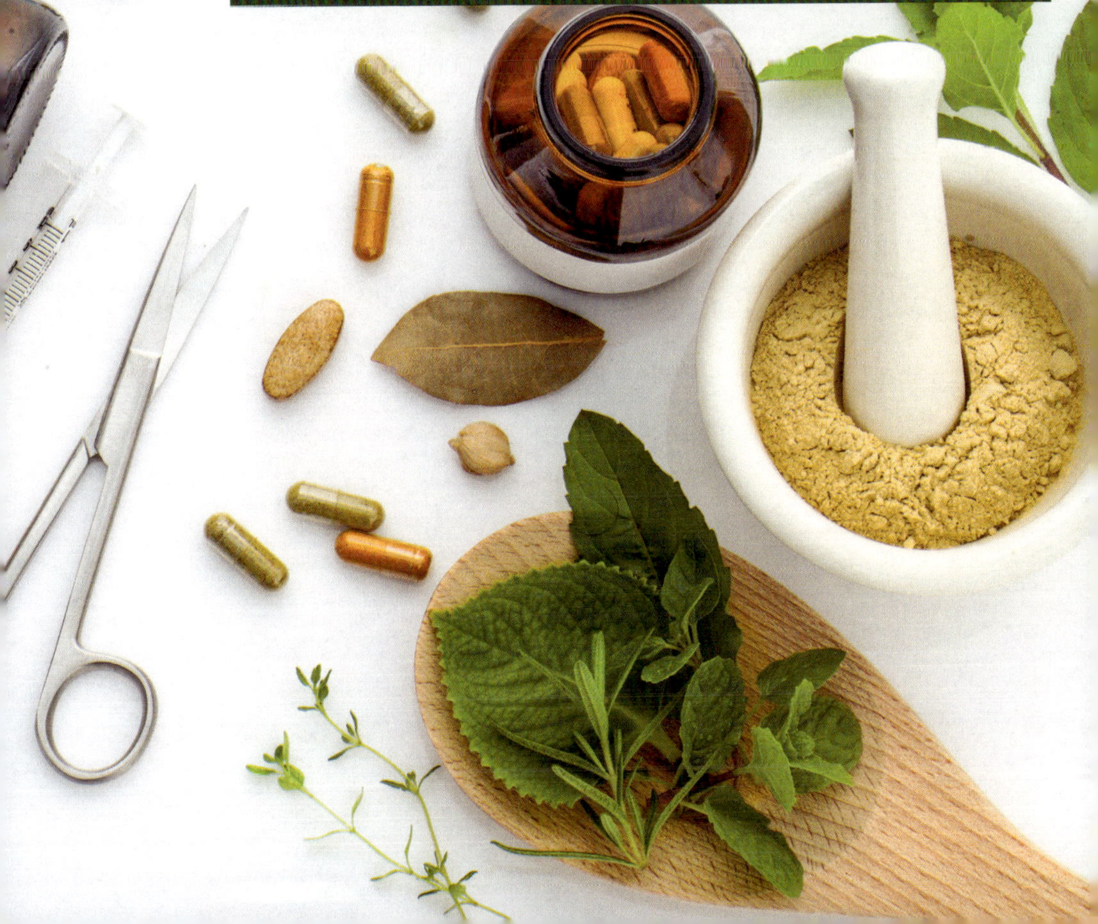

Sinister Solutions

Simple online searches make it incredibly easy for people to find sellers of alternative and natural medicines that make unproven claims. Unfortunately, many people are willing to take advantage of patients who are looking for anything they think will cure their cancer. The American Academy of Dermatology has reported on just a few of these alternative medicines and therapies that have been documented as being incredibly dangerous. In one example, in April 2017, the FDA warned 14 U.S.-based companies that sold fake cancer remedies to stop making false claims. These 14 companies illegally sold more than 65 products that they falsely claimed prevented, treated, and cured cancer. Using a fake remedy instead of seeking medical treatment delays the detection of skin cancer; by the time someone realizes their alternative treatment is not working, their cancer may have become much more difficult to treat.

Studies in Germany have found that using mistletoe as a treatment actually causes melanoma to spread more quickly, despite a belief by some that mistletoe boosts the body's immune system. Vitamins A and C in a patient's system can lead to serious complications if they are receiving radiation therapy or chemotherapy at the same time. In Australia, the government is warning people against the purchase and use of certain ointments, which are causing holes to develop on the skin months after application. One unfortunate person had part of his nose disappear after using a treatment known as black salve. He had initially refused a biopsy for a growth on his nose, preferring to treat it with what he thought was a safe, natural remedy.

Speaking with a doctor and dermatologist before beginning a treatment found online could very easily save someone from pain and disfigurement. Asking questions and researching credible resources are a person's best bet in finding an effective treatment that meets their needs.

Many Approaches, Many Practitioners

Patients who want to try a complementary or integrative approach may seek out help from an acupuncturist, a chiropractor, a naturopath, a homeopath, or any number of other practitioners. Acupuncturists frequently offer support to patients who are going through radiation therapy or chemotherapy. They work on the patient using a combination of massage, acupuncture—the insertion of many small, thin needles at certain pressure points—and sometimes herbs. The effectiveness of acupuncture is still being studied, but many patients who are experiencing side effects of chemotherapy or radiation, such as nausea, vomiting, pain, and shortness of breath, have reported improvement in their side-effect symptoms after trying acupuncture.

Chiropractors work to keep the body's nervous system healthy by manipulating the spine. Many also offer nutritional advice and suggest alternatives to drug treatment. Naturopathic doctors specialize in finding nutritional and herbal remedies to support a patient's recovery. Homeopathic practitioners believe in using diluted, or watered down, treatments to allow the body to heal itself. Some oncologists view alternative medicine with alarm, because few of these techniques have been verified or tested by medical doctors or the FDA. Most doctors, however, do not object to complementary techniques if they give the patient relief and do not interfere with the medications they are already taking. Most CAM treatments are not dangerous, and although their effectiveness is debatable, a patient who feels better after receiving an alternative treatment often does not care whether the improvement is all in their imagination.

With integrative medicine, conventional and complementary practitioners work together to make a patient more comfortable or to reduce the side effects that some patients experience. Some cancer treatment centers have made it easier for conventional and complementary practitioners to work together by establishing departments devoted to complementary medicine. For example, a chemotherapy patient at one of these centers might have an acupuncture treatment after their chemotherapy session to reduce the nausea chemotherapy often causes.

No matter what treatment strategy a patient chooses, it is more likely to work if the cancer has been

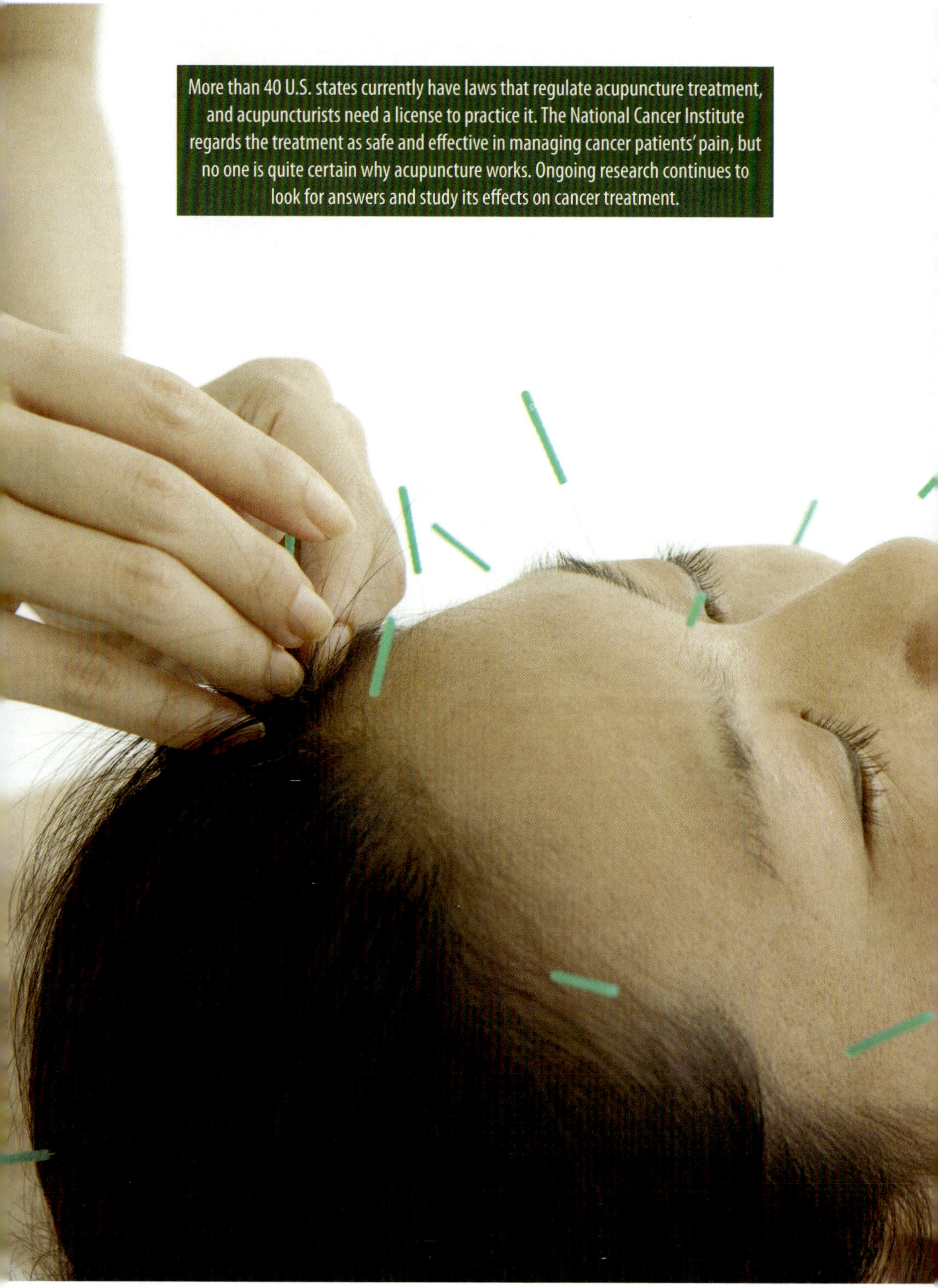

More than 40 U.S. states currently have laws that regulate acupuncture treatment, and acupuncturists need a license to practice it. The National Cancer Institute regards the treatment as safe and effective in managing cancer patients' pain, but no one is quite certain why acupuncture works. Ongoing research continues to look for answers and study its effects on cancer treatment.

caught at an early stage. Skin cancer patients sometimes feel frustrated because there is no single perfect treatment option. Their options, however, are always expanding. Researchers and oncologists are constantly working to develop new treatments for cancer as well as improve existing treatments to make them work faster and cause fewer side effects. After rigorous testing for safety and effectiveness, many of these new advances will eventually be approved for medical use.

CHAPTER SEVEN

CANCER RESEARCH: TODAY AND TOMORROW

Scientists and doctors are constantly investigating new approaches to treating cancer. They are applying new technologies to old problems, sometimes with surprising results. Some researchers are trying to develop a cancer vaccine, while others are applying DNA technology to try to find a way to help the body repair cells that have damaged DNA. Other studies are aiming to learn more about changes that occur in cancer cells, leading to new cancer-targeting drugs.

Volunteers Put to the Test

Cancer patients sometimes have the opportunity to try forms of treatment that are not yet approved by the FDA. Some cancer patients can volunteer to participate in clinical trials, in which they agree to test new forms of treatment. The way clinical trials work may vary depending on the disease and treatment being tested. Cancer-related clinical trials consist of five phases that need to be passed successfully before FDA approval; these phases ensure that that the tested treatment will be safe for general use.

Phase 0 is sometimes used at the beginning of a clinical trial. In this phase, researchers discover new treatments and test them for effectiveness and side effects. Sometimes cancer-fighting drugs do not do their intended jobs, so researchers need to know of any issues now rather than in future trial phases. Phase 0 is done with 15 or fewer participants, and the dose of the tested drug is so small that there is little risk in being a volunteer in this stage.

In Phase I of a clinical trial, researchers look for any potential side effects of the new drug in a group of up to a few dozen volunteers. The key here is finding a dosage that effectively treats cancer without having too many serious negative effects. Because the drug's side effects may not all be known at this time, doctors start by giving very low doses of the drug and monitoring patients closely. The main purpose of a Phase I trial is to find out whether a drug is safe by observing how the drug and the body interact with each other. If the drug is deemed relatively safe, the trial will move on to a bigger group.

In Phase II, 25 to 100 volunteers receive the highest safe dose determined in Phase I of the trial. Phase II is designed to determine whether the drug is effective in treating the targeted disease. Generally, the dosages are the same for all the volunteers, but some studies will observe differences in dosages and how the drug is administered. Phase I and Phase II are done in major cancer treatment centers, and no placebo groups—groups that are given fake treatments as a way to see how well the new drug works compared to no drug at all—are used.

Phase III is often the last phase of a trial that needs to be successful before a drug or treatment is approved for general use. Phase III aims to compare the effectiveness and safety of the new treatment with the current standard treatment. Several hundred participants are chosen and randomly assigned to receive either the new treatment or the standard treatment. Occasionally, placebos are used. Neither the patient nor their doctors will know which treatment was assigned, in an effort to determine which treatment is more effective. This is known as a double-blind study.

A new drug application is submitted to the FDA once the clinical trial is completed safely and effectively. If the results of the clinical trial were found to be more effective than the current standard treatment, the FDA will approve the new drug as the new standard treatment. However, if there are more questions or concerns, the FDA will ask for further studies and testing.

The FDA will continue to look at approved drugs and treatments over many years. This is known as Phase IV testing. This phase looks at

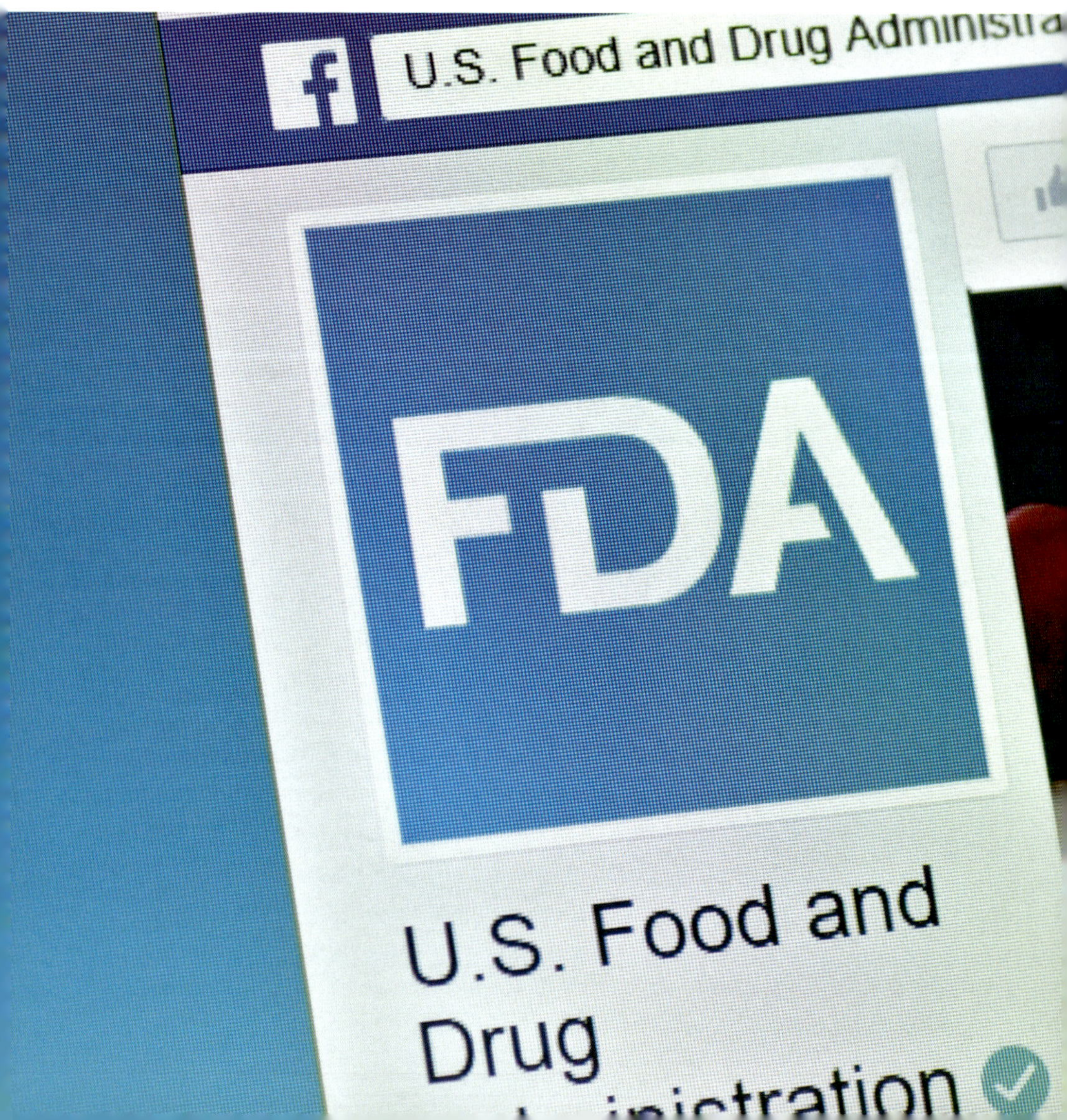

long-term side effects that may not have been seen in earlier phases, as well as the cost effectiveness of the drug and improvements in quality of life. This phase is done with thousands of participants and is considered the safest trial, as the drug has already been deemed safe for people to take. Phase IV studies are incredibly beneficial to researchers and future cancer patients, as they give people more information about a treatment's effectiveness and side effects and answer any remaining long-term questions.

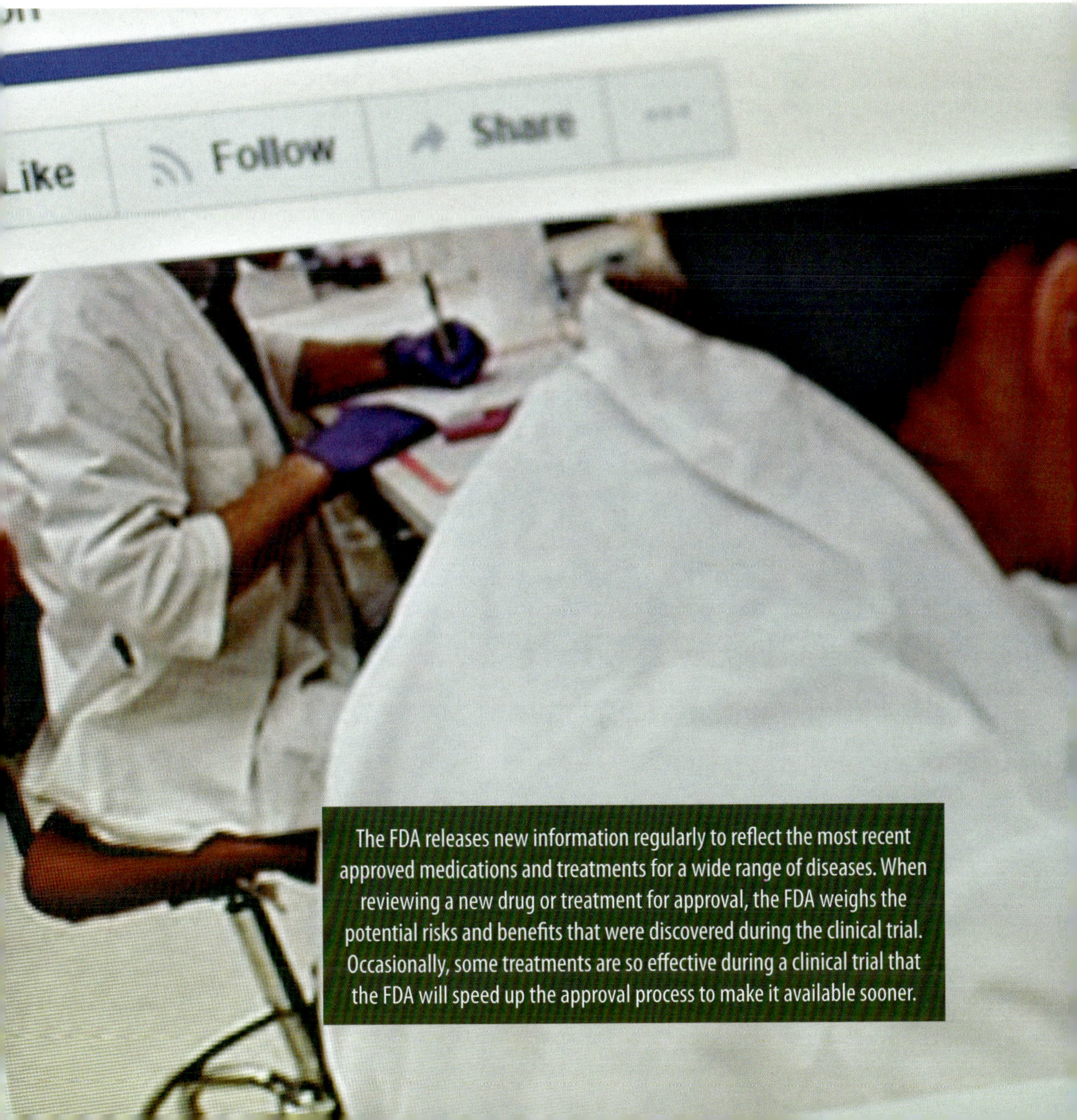

The FDA releases new information regularly to reflect the most recent approved medications and treatments for a wide range of diseases. When reviewing a new drug or treatment for approval, the FDA weighs the potential risks and benefits that were discovered during the clinical trial. Occasionally, some treatments are so effective during a clinical trial that the FDA will speed up the approval process to make it available sooner.

Adoptive Cell Immunotherapy

In 2018, after several ongoing clinical trials, the American Society of Clinical Oncology named adoptive cell immunotherapy the "clinical cancer advance of the year."[1] The clinical trials studied the effects of what are known as chimeric antigen receptor (CAR) T cells, or lab-engineered T cells. Immune cells in people's bodies search for intruder cells such as viruses and bacteria. The cells that fight off these intruders are known as T cells. Cancer cells, however, know how to hide from T cells and can go undetected—and unattacked—in the body. T cells, therefore, cannot detect or fight off cancer cells effectively.

Adoptive cell immunotherapy focuses on fighting cancer directly using CAR T cells, which were first developed in the late 1980s. This immunotherapy involves extracting white blood cells and T cells from a patient and adding an artificial gene in a laboratory. These added genes create CAR T cells. These engineered cells are then injected back into a patient's body, where they naturally multiply and get to work. The artificial gene that was added to the T cell allows for the new CAR T cells to detect, target, and attack cancer cells in the body. These cells have been found to be very successful in various clinical trials.

In August 2017, the FDA approved one CAR T-cell therapy based on its effectiveness against acute lymphocytic leukemia, or cancer of the blood and bone marrow, in children and young adults. Three months into its clinical trials, the CAR T-cell therapy made the leukemia go into remission in 82 percent of its participants, and six months later, 75 percent of the participants still had not relapsed. In adults, large B-cell lymphoma was also found to respond to adoptive cell immunotherapy. In one of those clinical studies, the use of CAR T cells had an 82 percent success rate against various lymphomas, with remission occurring in 54 percent of participants.

As with any new treatment or drug, not all side effects are currently known. Furthermore, the use of CAR T cells in adoptive cell immunotherapy has a range of serious and potentially dangerous side effects. Through further testing and research, doctors

An Experimental Treatment

Scientists are still learning how to replace a defective or missing gene in a damaged cell—something that is known as gene therapy. There are numerous gene therapy clinical studies being conducted. Typically, genetic material is introduced through a carrier, or vector, such as an inactive virus. This harmless virus will then carry genetic materials directly to the cells.

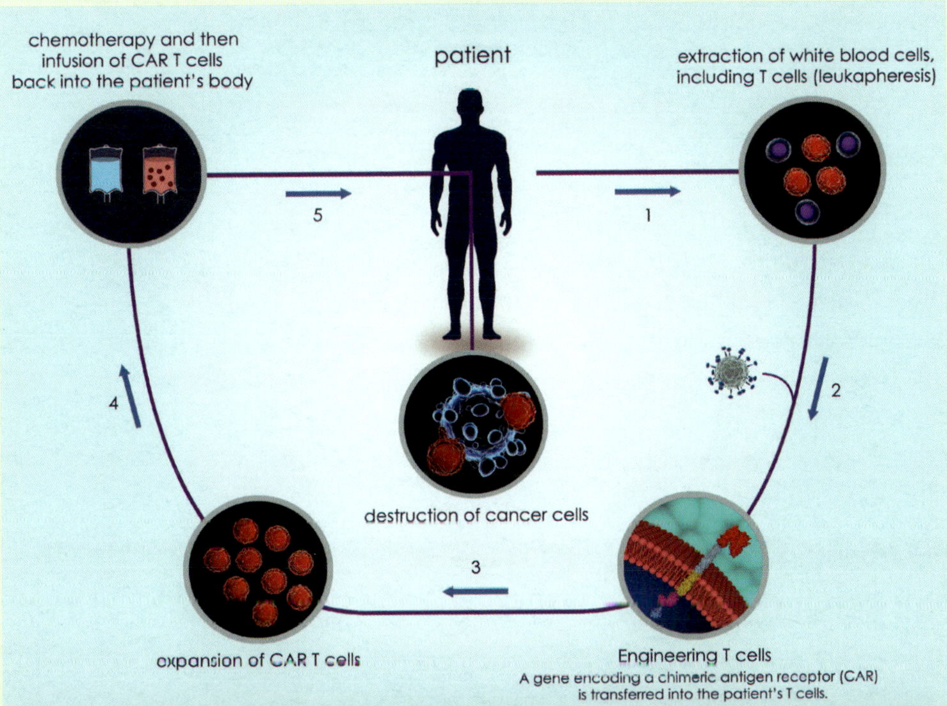

CAR T cells have been found to be effective against lymphoma, which is cancer of the immune system. In skin lymphoma, T cells multiply uncontrollably within the skin. This illustration demonstrates the basic steps of CAR T-cell therapy, which may continue to be found effective in treating many types of cancers.

and scientists have found ways to treat and even reverse some of the side effects. The use of adoptive cell immunotherapy has already had great success, and researchers are constantly working to improve its safety and effectiveness.

1. "Advance of the Year," American Society of Clinical Oncology, 2018. www.asco.org/research-progress/reports-studies/clinical-cancer-advances-2018/advance-year.

The purpose of gene therapy is to create and repair cells that can detect, target, and hopefully destroy cancer cells directly. Tumor suppressor genes have been designed to prevent tumor growth and cancer regression. Another type of gene therapy aims to make cancer cells more sensitive to radiation and chemotherapy treatments, making these treatments more effective.

Researchers are even inserting genes that reverse and lessen the side effects of cancer treatments. There are several types of gene therapies, and all of them are being studied closely.

Because gene therapy is still relatively new, it is considered an experimental treatment. This is why clinical trials and studies are so crucial at this point. Gene therapy has its drawbacks, just like any other cancer treatment. For instance, flu-like symptoms are sometimes seen in patients who have received gene therapy. Furthermore, the use and creation of too many modified genes in the body, known as overexpression, can lead to more cancer development. Gene therapy can also be accidentally introduced into healthy cells, leading to other complications.

The Sunscreen Gene

Some people seem to have a natural resistance to skin cancer, and as it turns out, there is actually a gene that makes this possible. The gene, first discovered in the 1990s, is known as UVRAG, or UV radiation resistance-associated gene. DNA cell damage occurs immediately after UV ray exposure, and those people with a healthy version of UVRAG have some of this damage repaired. It has been observed in at least one study, however, that those with lower levels or mutated versions of UVRAG had cancer spread more easily in their bodies. They also had lower survival rates compared to those who had better levels of the resistance gene.

It is important to note, though, that this gene does not have miracle properties. Skin cancer is still a possibility for anyone exposed to UV rays. The presence of healthy UVRAGs simply means that the body can better handle DNA cell damage. The gene itself suppresses tumor development, helping to prevent cancer from forming and spreading. Taking proper precautions against damaging UV rays is still a person's best bet in preventing skin cancer from developing.

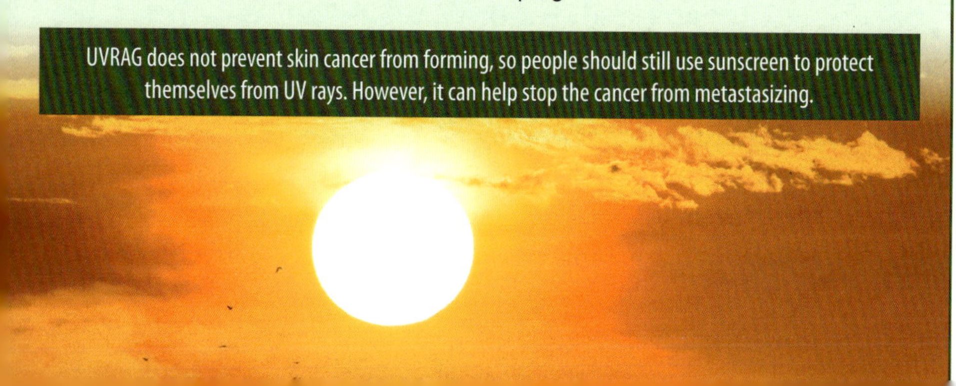

UVRAG does not prevent skin cancer from forming, so people should still use sunscreen to protect themselves from UV rays. However, it can help stop the cancer from metastasizing.

Enzymes That Stop Cancer

Some skin cancer researchers have focused on trying to understand what causes cancer to metastasize. In 2005, researchers announced the results of a study of an enzyme called focal adhesion kinase (FAK), which is present in skin cancer cells. The study's authors found that FAK is overactive in skin cancers and that FAK activity triggers the cancer to spread. They hypothesized that treatments targeting this enzyme could stop cancer cells from traveling throughout the body. In the lab, they discovered that if they disrupted FAK activity in aggressive cancer cells, the cells' ability to metastasize dropped by 70 percent.

In September 2017, researchers at the University of Pennsylvania School of Medicine targeted an enzyme that is responsible for tumor growth and tumor protection. With these findings, new drugs were tested in mice that stopped melanoma and pancreatic tumor growth. Previous FDA-approved drugs that were meant to stop tumor growth also unintentionally made the tumor resistant to treatment. This study was able to find an enzyme that effectively solved both problems, stopping the tumor both from growing and from repairing itself. These findings will undoubtedly lead to more advancements in the future.

A Skin to Heal All Wounds

Fortunately, most skin cancer patients do not face a struggle with cancer cells that are metastasizing throughout their body. Instead, many face a more everyday concern: avoiding disfigurement by their treatment. Repeated surgeries can leave a patient with multiple scars. Some patients lose so much skin that it is not possible for surgeons to sew the wound together. In the past, this meant they would have to take skin

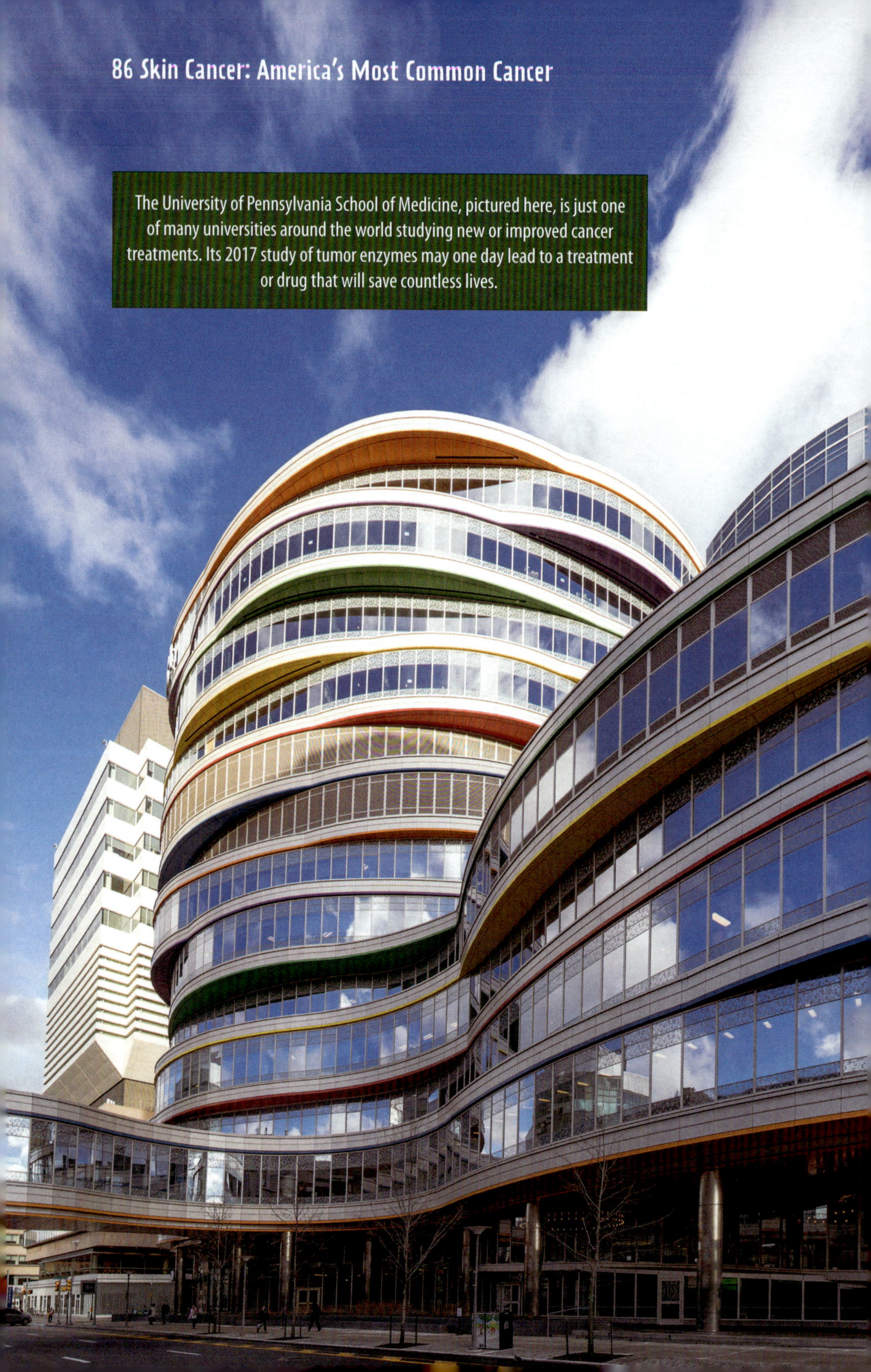

The University of Pennsylvania School of Medicine, pictured here, is just one of many universities around the world studying new or improved cancer treatments. Its 2017 study of tumor enzymes may one day lead to a treatment or drug that will save countless lives.

grafts from another part of the body. Having a graft of their own skin is still an option for skin cancer patients. In this process, a piece of skin from a more hidden part of the body, such as the upper thigh, is cut off and moved to the part of the body that is being treated for skin cancer.

Bioengineers, however, have been able to produce different kinds of artificial skin since the 1970s. A professor and director of a burn treatment unit in a Massachusetts hospital first developed an artificial skin using shark cartilage and cowhide collagen. According to the Massachusetts General Hospital Burn Research Center, "Every similar artificial skin product that has since been researched and developed hinges upon the conceptual framework that eventually yielded this artificial skin system."[34]

Some artificial skins are being developed to treat burn patients, skin cancer patients, and others who have serious skin conditions. It is even being applied to artificial limbs to give patients back their sense of touch. Some of these skins can actually sense temperature, and in January 2017, engineers from the California Institute of Technology reported a new advancement in this technology. Using an everyday food product known as pectin, the researchers developed a skin that can better detect temperature changes. Other artificial skins are being developed that can heal themselves.

In February 2018, researchers from Stanford University announced even better artificial skin advancements. According to engineer Zhenan Bao, "Research into synthetic skin and flexible electronics has come a long way, but until now no one had demonstrated a process to reliably manufacture stretchable circuits."[35] These circuits can allow patients to feel something as gentle as a ladybug crawling over their hands. There are many possible applications for artificial skin, and scientists are working to make this skin look and act as real as possible. The cost of technology and manufacturing is one of the biggest roadblocks at the moment, so research is ongoing.

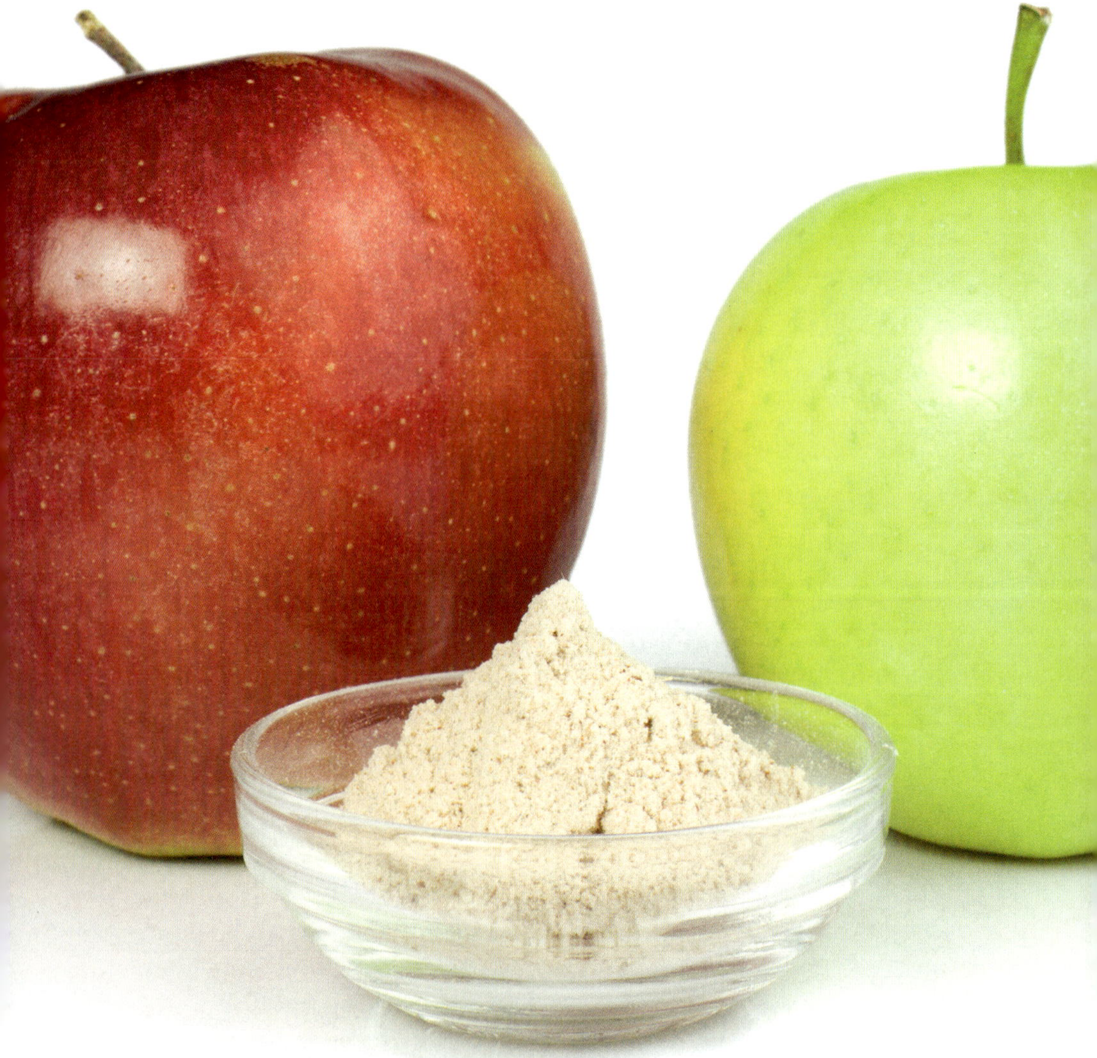

Pectin is a carbohydrate that comes from fruits, and it is responsible for keeping a fruit ripe and firm. In its powdered form (shown here), it is used as a gelling agent. In 2017, researchers used pectin in their creation of an artificial skin that could sense changes in temperature.

Skin cancer treatment continues to improve every year as new advancements are made and new drugs and treatments are approved. Surviving skin cancer, however, does not rely on treatment alone. The biggest factor in skin cancer survival is detecting and removing it early. Prevention is still the best policy: People of all ages around the world should take every precaution in regard to UV protection.

When detected early enough, skin cancers are often completely treatable, and survival rates for more serious types of skin cancers, though far from perfect, continue to improve. Years of trial and error and potentially huge advancements lie ahead.

NOTES

Introduction: Thinking Twice About the Sun

1. Quoted in Cassie Shortsleeve, "Why Melanoma Isn't the Only Kind of Skin Cancer You Need to Worry About," *Men's Health*, May 24, 2016. www.thedermatologygroup.com/blog/index.php/why-melanoma-isnt-the-only-kind-of-skin-cancer-you-need-to-worry-about.
2. Lawrence E. Gibson, M.D., "Tanning: Does a Base Tan Prevent Sunburn?," Mayo Clinic, July 11, 2017. www.mayoclinic.org/diseases-conditions/sunburn/expert-answers/tanning/faq-20057866.
3. Stacey Simon, "The Ugly Truth About Indoor Tanning," American Cancer Society, May 1, 2015. www.cancer.org/latest-news/the-ugly-truth-about-indoor-tanning.html.
4. "Study: Most Americans Don't Use Sunscreen," American Academy of Dermatology, May 19, 2015. www.aad.org/media/news-releases/study-most-americans-don-t-use-sunscreen.
5. "Protecting Children from Ultraviolet Radiation," World Health Organization, December 11, 2009. www.who.int/uv/resources/archives/fs261/en.
6. "Skin Cancer Facts and Statistics," Skin Cancer Foundation, January 31, 2018. www.skincancer.org/skin-cancer-information/skin-cancer-facts.
7. Dr. H. William Higgins II and Dr. David Leffell, "Melanoma at Its Most Curable," Skin Cancer Foundation, May 4, 2016. www.skincancer.org/skin-cancer-information/melanoma/in-situ.

Chapter One: Defining Skin Cancer

8. Gregory L. Wells, "Basal Cell Carcinoma," *Merck Manuals*, accessed on April 23, 2018. www.merckmanuals.com/home/skin-disorders/skin-cancers/basal-cell-carcinoma.

9. Quoted in "Study: Most Americans Don't Use Sunscreen," American Academy of Dermatology.
10. "Sun Safety," Centers for Disease Control and Prevention, June 13, 2017. www.cdc.gov/cancer/skin/basic_info/sun-safety.htm.
11. Quoted in "Study: Most Americans Don't Use Sunscreen," American Academy of Dermatology.
12. Daniel J. DeNoon, "The Truth About Vitamin D: Why You Need Vitamin D," WebMD, November 30, 2010. www.webmd.com/osteoporosis/features/the-truth-about-vitamin-d-why-you-need-vitamin-d.
13. Anne Marie McNeill, "Skin Cancer and Vitamin D," *The Skin Cancer Foundation Journal*, May 18, 2016. www.skincancer.org/healthy-lifestyle/vitamin-d/damage.
14. "Diet and Physical Activity: What's the Cancer Connection?," American Cancer Society, April 14, 2017. www.cancer.org/cancer/cancer-causes/diet-physical-activity/diet-and-physical-activity.html.

Chapter Two: A Growing Cause for Concern

15. "Key Statistics for Melanoma Skin Cancer," American Cancer Society, January 4, 2018. www.cancer.org/cancer/melanoma-skin-cancer/about/key-statistics.html.
16. Maritza Perez, "Ask the Expert: Can Darker Skinned People Get Skin Cancer?," Skin Cancer Foundation, 2009. www.skincancer.org/skin-cancer-information/ask-the-experts/can-darker-skinned-people-get-skin-cancer.
17. "Melanoma Cancer Risk," National Cancer Institute, September 10, 2008. www.cancer.gov/melanomarisktool/melanoma-cancer-risk.html.
18. "Basal and Squamous Cell Skin Cancer Risk Factors," American Cancer Society, May 10, 2016. www.cancer.org/cancer/basal-and-squamous-cell-skin-cancer/causes-risks-prevention/risk-factors.html.

19. "Skin Cancer," Cancer Council Australia, last updated May 21, 2018. www.cancer.org.au/about-cancer/types-of-cancer/skin-cancer.html.
20. "Basal and Squamous Cell Skin Cancer Risk Factors," American Cancer Society.
21. Quoted in "Summer Sanders' New Direction," Skin Cancer Foundation, May 19, 2017. www.skincancer.org/true-stories/summer-sanders.

Chapter Four: Common Carcinomas

22. "Key Statistics for Basal and Squamous Cell Skin Cancer," American Cancer Society, January 4, 2018. www.cancer.org/cancer/basal-and-squamous-cell-skin-cancer/about/key-statistics.html.
23. Erika Stalder, "Here's What You Need to Know About UVC Rays," *Refinery29*, March 31, 2014. www.refinery29.com/2014/03/65328/uvc-rays.
24. "Health Effects of UV Radiation," United States Environmental Protection Agency, accessed on April 24, 2018. www.epa.gov/sunsafety/health-effects-uv-radiation.
25. Quoted in Dean Monti, "A Reporter's Fight Against Skin Cancer," *Dermatology Insights*, vol. 3, no. 2., 2002, p. 18. www.skinident.es/fileadmin/img/spanish-pictures/pdf/Dermatology_Insights_2.pdf.
26. "Risk Factors for Anal Cancer," American Cancer Society, November 13, 2017. www.cancer.org/cancer/anal-cancer/causes-risks-prevention/risk-factors.html.
27. "Skin Cancer—Squamous Cell Carcinoma," The Angeles Clinic, accessed on April 24, 2018. www.theangelesclinic.org/Home/PatientEducationLibrary/tabid/19283/ctl/View/mid/35200/Default.aspx?ContentPubID=354.

Chapter Five: Rare, Deadly, and Steady

28. "Cancer Stat Facts: Melanoma of the Skin," National Cancer Institute, accessed on April 24, 2018. seer.cancer.gov/statfacts/html/melan.html.

29. "Melanoma Facts and Statistics," Melanoma Research Foundation, accessed on April 24, 2018. www.melanoma.org/understand-melanoma/what-melanoma/melanoma-facts-and-stats.

30. "Five or More Blistering Sunburns Before Age 20 May Increase Melanoma Risk by 80 Percent," American Association for Cancer Research, May 29, 2014. www.aacr.org/Newsroom/Pages/News-Release-Detail.aspx?ItemID=553#.WtFZPfnwaUl.

31. "Melanoma Risk Factors," AIM at Melanoma Foundation, accessed on April 24, 2018. www.aimatmelanoma.org/melanoma-risk-factors.

32. "Melanoma Stats, Facts, and Figures," AIM at Melanoma Foundation, accessed on April 24, 2018. www.aimatmelanoma.org/about-melanoma/melanoma-stats-facts-and-figures.

33. Jamie Troil Goldfarb, "Survivor Stories," Melanoma Research Alliance, accessed on April 24, 2018. www.curemelanoma.org/about-melanoma/melanoma-stories/survivor-stories.

Chapter Seven: Cancer Research: Today and Tomorrow

34. "The Development of Artificial Skin," MGH Burn Research Center, accessed on April 25, 2018. www.burnresearchcenter.org/brcpublicwebsite/artificialskin.htm.

35. Quoted in Andrew Myers and Tom Abate, "Stanford Researchers Develop Stretchable, Touch-Sensitive Electronics," *Stanford News*, February 19, 2018. news.stanford.edu/press-releases/2018/02/19/stretchable-touctive-electronics.

GLOSSARY

ABCDE test: A way to screen for skin cancer by checking for asymmetry, border irregularity, color variation, diameter, and elevation of moles.

benign: Unlikely to spread or cause harm.

biopsy: A kind of surgery in which a doctor takes a sample of tissue for examination.

dermatologist: A doctor who specializes in skin disorders.

DNA: The genetic material in a cell.

dysplastic nevi: Unusual-looking moles.

immunotherapy: Therapy that works by stimulating the body's immune system.

malignant: Likely to spread and potentially deadly.

melanocyte: A pigment-producing skin cell.

melanoma: A cancer that develops from a melanocyte.

metastasis: When a cancer spreads from its original site to other parts of the body.

nonmelanoma: A skin cancer that is not a melanoma; one that develops out of the basal or squamous cells.

oncologist: A doctor who specializes in treating cancer.

photodynamic therapy: A type of therapy in which a tumor is treated with light-sensitive drugs and then subjected to intense light. The light activates the drugs, killing the cancer cells but leaving normal skin unharmed.

topical: Applied to the surface of the skin, instead of being taken by mouth or injected.

ORGANIZATIONS TO CONTACT

AIM at Melanoma Foundation
3217 Bob O Link Court
Plano, TX 75093
(916) 706-0599
www.aimatmelanoma.org
The AIM at Melanoma Foundation works to pursue legislation and K–12 education regarding the dangers of indoor tanning by minors. The website provides information for melanoma patients and their families as well as information about global research initiatives.

The American Academy of Dermatology (AAD)
P.O. Box 1968
Des Plaines, IL 60017
(888) 462-3376
www.aad.org
The American Academy of Dermatology's website provides tips and information regarding a variety of skin conditions and possible treatments. It also includes dermatologist and skin screening locations that users can search for by state and city.

American Cancer Society (ACS)
250 Williams Street NW
Atlanta, GA 30303
(800) 227-2345
www.cancer.org
The American Cancer Society's website provides in-depth information and resources that cover a wide range of cancer topics, as well as current research and statistics. The ACS even offers a Cancer Helpline and live chat as well as local support locations.

National Cancer Institute (NCI)
BG 9609 MSC 9760
9609 Medical Center Drive
Bethesda, MD 20892-9760
(800) 422-6237
www.cancer.gov
The National Cancer Institute, founded in 1937, continues to educate the American public on cancer. Its website addresses numerous topics, such as cancer stages, coping skills for patients, and a long list of cancer support services that cover a variety of needs.

The Skin Cancer Foundation
205 Lexington Avenue, 11th Floor
New York, NY 10016
(212) 725-5176
www.skincancer.org
The Skin Cancer Foundation educates the public about skin cancer warning signs, prevention, and treatment options. It also offers survivor stories, the organization's approved list of UV-protection products, and a physician locator.

FOR MORE INFORMATION

Books

Esposito, Lisa. *Cancer Information for Teens*. Boston, MA: Credo Reference, 2014.
This book includes several chapters on skin cancer and includes information about coping with cancer at home and at school, as well as tips on how to support a friend or family member who has cancer.

Grayzel, Eva. *You Are Not Alone: Families Touched by Cancer*. Talk4Hope Books, 2010.
Using stories from children from around the world who have been affected by cancer in some way, this book is meant to help readers cope with and discuss cancer diagnoses within their families.

National Cancer Institute. *When Your Parent Has Cancer: A Guide for Teens*. CreateSpace Independent Publishing Platform, 2012.
This book provides readers with stories from teenagers who have experienced life with a parent who has cancer. It also helps teen readers locate support groups.

New York State Department of Health. *Skin Cancer: Cause and Cure (A Concise Guide to Skin Cancer)*. CreateSpace Independent Publishing Platform, 2014.
Written with the assistance of organizations such as the CDC and NCI, this book provides information on screening techniques, risk factors, and treatment options.

Stanley, David L. *Melanoma: It Started with a Freckle*. McGann Publishing LLC, 2016.
In this memoir, author David Stanley explains his life and battle with melanoma, inspiring readers to face similar health issues with heart and humor.

Websites

American Society for Dermatologic Surgery (ASDS)
www.asds.net
The ASDS website provides resources on skin care, free cancer screening locations, and a dermatologist locator.

Centers for Disease Control and Prevention: Skin Cancer
www.cdc.gov/cancer/skin
This section of the CDC website covers news and statistics on skin cancer in the United States as well as offering tips on prevention and treatment.

Melanoma Research Foundation
www.melanoma.org
This nonprofit organization advocates for melanoma research and provides an online forum for melanoma patients. Always ask a parent or guardian before participating in an online forum.

Science Daily
www.sciencedaily.com
This website features the latest news and research developments on a wide range of various health topics, including skin cancer.

SkinCancer.net
www.skincancer.net
This website offers information on skin cancer, articles from medical professionals, and survivor stories. It uses only credible sources, such as the FDA and the ACS.

INDEX

M

N

P

S

T

U

V

W

PICTURE CREDITS

Cover (main) BSIP/Getty Images; cover, back cover, pp. 1–6, 10–11, 18, 20, 26, 29, 34, 36, 39, 42, 47, 51, 54, 60, 64, 66, 69, 74, 78, 82–84, 90, 94–95, 97, 99, 103–104 (green texture) foxaon1987/Shutterstock.com; back cover (texture) Evannovostro/Shutterstock.com; p. 7 Evgeniy Kalinovskiy/Shutterstock.com; p. 8 Rido/Shutterstock.com; pp. 9, 44 gritsalak karalak/Shutterstock.com; pp. 11, 12, 28, 36 Designua/Shutterstock.com; p. 13 jax10289/Shutterstock.com; p. 15 Nadezhda1906/iStock/Thinkstock; p. 17 bitt24/Shutterstock.com; pp. 18–19 Umpaporn/Shutterstock.com; pp. 22–23 adriaticfoto/Shutterstock.com; p. 25 xavierarnau/iStock Unreleased/Getty Images; pp. 30–31 Andrey_Popov/Shutterstock.com; p. 32 Rob Bayer/Shutterstock.com; p. 38 JodiJacobson/E+/Getty Images; p. 40 Geo-grafika/Shutterstock.com; p. 46 Brandon Tabiolo/Perspectives/Getty Images; p. 49 BonD80/Shutterstock.com; p. 57 ViewStock/Getty Images; p. 58 Burger/Canopy/Getty Images; p. 62 Alfred Pasieka/Science Photo Library/Getty Images; p. 67 Blamb/Shutterstock.com; p. 68 Constantine Pankin/Shutterstock.com; pp. 70–71 BrianAJackson/iStock/Thinkstock; pp. 72–73 Kerdkanno/Shutterstock.com; p. 76 Leonardo da/Shutterstock.com; pp. 80–81 g0d4ather/Shutterstock.com; p. 83 Meletios Verras/Shutterstock.com; p. 84 Happy Together/Shutterstock.com; p. 86 SINITAR/Shutterstock.com; p. 88 Deyan Georgiev/Shutterstock.com.

ABOUT THE AUTHOR

Peter Kogler is currently a schoolteacher in Buffalo, New York. When he is not teaching, he loves to write, collect old toys, and read everything he can get his hands on. He especially loves to read about current events and breakthroughs in the medical and science fields. This is his second educational book, and it is one that is very important to him. His father, who worked outside for years, was recently diagnosed with skin cancer. He wrote this book to give answers, hope, and inspiration to those readers who need it most.